Progress in Pediatric Hematology/Oncology, Volume II

BONE TUMORS
IN
CHILDREN

Norman Jaffe, M.B. Bch., Dip. Paed.
Professor of Pediatrics, University of Texas Cancer Center
Division Chief, Division of Solid Tumors
M.D. Anderson Hospital and Tumor Institute
Houston, Texas

Carl Pochedly, M.D.
Denis R. Miller, M.D.
Series Editors

RC280
B6
B68
1979

PSG Publishing Company, Inc.
Littleton, Massachusetts

349433

Library of Congress Cataloging in Publication Data
Main entry under title:

Bone tumors in children.

    (Progress in pediatric hematology/oncology ; v. 2)
    Includes index.
    1.   Bones—Tumors.   2.   Tumors in Children.
I.   Jaffe, Norman.   II.   Series. [DNLM: 1.   Bone
neoplasma—In infancy and childhood.   W1PR677E v. 2 /
WE258 B7121]
RC280.B6B68   618.9′29′9471   77-94881
ISBN 0-88416-142-0

Printed in the United States of America.

International Standard Book Number: 0-88416-142-0

International Standard Book Series Number: 0-88416-136-6

Library of Congress Catalog Card Number: 77-94881

To my wife, Louise

In preparing this book

her love inspired me

her patience sustained me.

EDITORS AND CONTRIBUTORS

Progress in Pediatric Hematology/Oncology
Volume II
BONE TUMORS IN CHILDREN

Series Editors

Carl Pochedly, M.D.
Denis R. Miller, M.D.

Contributors to this Volume

Norman Jaffe, M.B. Bch.,
  Dip. Paed.
Professor of Pediatrics
University of Texas
  Cancer Center
Division Chief, Division of
  Solid Tumors
M.D. Anderson Hospital &
  Tumor Institute
Houston, Texas

John G. Camblin, M.D.
Staff Physician, Orthopedics
  Section
Veterans Administration
  Hospital
Instructor, Department of
  Orthopedics
College of Medicine
University of Florida
Gainesville, Florida

J. Robert Cassady, M.D.
Associate Professor of
  Radiation Therapy
Harvard Medical School
Radiotherapist, Joint Center
  for Radiation Therapy
Children's Hospital Medical
  Center
Boston, Massachusetts

David C. Dahlin, M.D.
Chairman, Department of
  Surgical Pathology
Mayo Clinic and Mayo
  Foundation
Professor of Pathology
Mayo Medical School
Rochester, Minnesota

Frederick R. Eilber, M.D.
Associate Professor of
  Surgery
Division of Oncology
School of Medicine
University of California
Los Angeles, California

William F. Enneking, M.D.
Professor and Chairman
Department of Othopedics
College of Medicine
University of Florida
Gainsville, Florida

Robert M. Filler, M.D.
Surgeon-in-Chief
Hospital for Sick Children
Professor of Surgery
University of Toronto
Toronto, Ontario, Canada
Formerly Chief of Clinical
  Surgery
Children's Hospital
  Medical Center and
Associate Professor of
  Surgery
Harvard Medical School
Boston, Massachusetts

Todd T. Grant, M.D.
Assistant Professor of
  Othopedic Surgery
Division of Orthopedics
Department of Surgery
School of Medicine
University of California
Los Angeles, California

Sydney Heyman, M.D.
Nuclear Radiologist
Children's Hospital
  Medical Center
Instructor of Radiology
Harvard Medical School
Boston, Massachusetts

Ronald B. Irwin, M.D.
Resident in Orthopedics
  (Oncology)
Mayo Graduate School of
  Medicine University of
  Minnesota
Rochester, Minnesota

John A. Kirkpatrick, M.D.
Radiologist-in-Chief
Children's Hospital Medical
  Center
Professor of Radiology
Harvard Medical School
Boston, Massachusetts

Ralph C. Marcove, M.D.
Chief, Bone Tumor Service
Hospital for Joint Diseases
Associate Attending at
  Memorial Sloan-Kettering
  Cancer Center and the
  Hospital for Special Surgery
Clinical Associate Professor
  of Surgery
Cornell University Medical
  College
New York, New York

Donald L. Morton, M.D.
Associate Professor of Surgery
Division of Oncology
School of Medicine
University of California
Los Angeles, California

Antoinette L. Pieroni, ACSW
Chief Social Worker
Sidney Farber Cancer Institute
Boston, Massachusetts

Gerald Rosen, M.D.
Attending Pediatrician,
  Department of Pediatrics
Memorial Sloan-Kettering
  Cancer Center
New York, New York

Fritz Schajowicz, M.D.
Professor of Pathology
Faculty of Medicine
University of Buenos Aires
Italian Hospital
Buenos Aires, Argentina

Franklin H. Sim, M.D.
Consultant, Department of
    Orthopedics
Mayo Clinic and Mayo
    Foundation
Assistant Professor of
    Orthopedic Surgery
Mayo Medical School
Rochester, Minnesota

Wataru W. Sutow, M.D.
Pediatrician, M.D. Anderson
    Hospital & Tumor Institute
Professor of Pediatrics
University of Texas System
    Cancer Center
Houston, Texas

Salvador Treves, M.D.
Chief, Pediatric Nuclear
    Medicine
Children's Hospital Medical
    Center
Instructor of Radiology
Harvard Medical School
Boston, Massachusetts

Hugh Watts, M.D.
Assistant Professor in
    Orthopedics
Harvard Medical School
Associate in Orthopedic
    Surgery
Children's Hospital Medical
    Center
Boston, Massachusetts

Ralph R. Weichselbaum, M.D.
Assistant Professor of
    Radiation Therapy
Harvard Medical School
Radiotherapist, Joint Center
    for Radiation Therapy
Radiotherapist
Peter Bent Brigham
    Hospital
Boston, Massachusetts

Robert H. Wilkinson, M.D.
Radiologist
Children's Hospital Medical
    Center
Associate Professor of
Radiology
Harvard Medical School
Boston, Massachusetts

CONTENTS

Bone cancer serves as a prototype for the coordinated multi-disciplinary treatment of malignancy. Such treatment is essential if optimum results are to be achieved. Therapy also must be carefully integrated since occasionally concepts appear as opposing forces. This is not unexpected since the "correct" treatment for most cancers is by no means firmly established. A fundamental principle, however, is that the plan of management must be sufficiently flexible to accommodate changing circumstances.

No attempt has been made to disguise controversies or differences of opinion. These emerged on a number of occasions between contributors and myself and, indeed, are known to exist among other contributors. This is illustrated particularly in the growing interest in limb preservation for osteosarcoma where diverse approaches center on operative technique, types of endoprostheses and use of preoperative chemotherapy and radiation therapy. This manual is replete with such diversities — an inevitable consequence of new discoveries and innovative changes.

Whenever concepts could not be resolved, authors were permitted wide discretion to express their own views. This resulted in some degree of overlap and duplication. However, it is precisely in the differences and diverse opinions that the strength of this work must lie. Inevitably, contemporary forms of treatment will be provided but the controversy surrounding such treatment must provoke vigorous stimuli to improve the results and prevent complications.

The responsibility of weighing the decision, examining the controversy and implementing treatment is assumed by the primary physician. He must serve as a patient's anchor to windward and often support his charge through a perilous journey. To alleviate his burden, this book has summoned assistance from the accumulated experience of investigators from diverse disciplines. It is in this spirit that I express a sense of deep gratitude to my distinguished colleagues and contributors without whose help and expertise this work would not have materialized.

Norman Jaffe

And He said unto me:
Son of man, can these bones live?
And I answered: O Lord God,
Thou knowest.

Ezekiel, Chapter 37

1 Malignant Bone Tumors in Children: Incidence and Etiologic Considerations

Norman Jaffe, M.B.Bch., Dip.Paed.

1. Host factors
   a. Growth
   b. Sex
   c. Metabolism
   d. Familial and genetic factors
   e. Ethnic factors
   f. Immune defects
   g. Target cell
2. Environmental factors
   a. Viruses
   b. Trauma
   c. Ionizing radiation
   d. Chemicals

Cancer ranks second behind accidents as the most common cause of death in children under 14 years of age.[1][2] Among cancers, the malignant bone tumors are relatively rare, occurring sixth in general incidence and in the following order: leukemia, tumors of the central nervous system, tumors of lymphoid tissue, neuroblastoma, Wilms' tumor, bone cancer, rhabdomyosarcoma, and retinoblastoma. Table 1 adapted from the Third National Cancer Survey, depicts the incidence of malignant tumors in 1,925 white children diagnosed between 1969 and 1971.[3] A similar incidence was observed in 225 black children.

The etiology of the skeletal sarcomas is unknown. Speculation draws primarily on factors derived from exogenous sources, particularly radiation therapy or viruses acting on host factors, but genetic influences must also be considered.

Investigations reported in this chapter were supported in part by research grant CA-06516 from the National Cancer Institute and by grant RR-05526 from the Division of Research Facilities and Resources, National Institutes of Health.

Table 1
Malignant Neoplasms in White Children under Fifteen Years of Age in the United States

Diagnosis	No. of Cases	Rate*
Leukemia	651	42.1
Lymphoma	204	13.2
Central nervous system	370	23.9
Sympathetic nervous system	148	9.6
Neuroblastoma	123	
Other	25	
Retinoblastoma	52	3.4
Kidney tumor	121	7.8
Wilms' tumor	117	
Other	4	
Liver tumor	29	1.9
Bone tumor	86	5.6
Osteosarcoma	51	
Ewing's sarcoma	26	
Other	9	
Gonadal and germ cell tumors	34	2.2
Ovary	17	
Testis	16	
Other	1	
Teratoma, nongonadal	5	0.3
Soft tissue tumors	130	8.4
Rhabdomyosarcoma	69	
Other	61	
Melanoma	11	0.7
Miscellaneous	84	5.4
Total	1,925	124.5

Adapted from Young and Miller.[3]
*Rates per million per year based on 1970 survey-area population of 5,151,699. Total U.S. 1970 population of white children under 15 years of age was 49,001,683.

HOST FACTORS

Growth

Osteosarcoma appears more commonly at the growing ends of bones and appears to be closely related to bone growth. This has been observed in dogs, where the relative risk of osteosarcoma in giant breeds such as the St. Bernard and Great Dane is approximately 200 times that for small- or medium-sized breeds, and a similar pattern has been detected in humans.[4-8] The incidence of osteosarcoma in humans appears to peak in two age groups. The first peak is in the 10- to 20-year-old age group, coinciding with the pubertal growth spurt. The second occurs at a more advanced age and may possibly be related to incidence of Paget's disease.

Sex

Osteosarcoma is distinctly more common in males, and this may also be related to bone growth. Average heights, by individual years of age, for boys and girls are similar (although the pubertal growth spurt in females has a somewhat earlier onset, and this may account for the earlier appearance of bone tumors in girls). Also until the age of 13, mortality rates from bone cancer are virtually identical for both sexes. After age 13, however, boys grow taller than girls, and the mortality rate for boys exceeds that for girls.[6]

Metabolism

Several studies have revealed abnormalities in carbohydrate metabolism and in insulin and somatomedin levels in patients with osteosarcoma.[9][10] Two abnormal patterns of glucose metabolism have been detected. The first is reflected by a glucose tolerance curve which is compatible with "chemical diabetes" coupled with hyperinsulinism. This was noted in patients with active disease. Reversion of the abnormal carbohydrate patterns to normal accompanied arrest of the tumor. High levels of somatomedin were also found. The latter is inhibited by estradiol, and since estrogens have been used to arrest linear growth in females, their therapeutic use in osteosarcoma was also considered.

The second pattern involved development of hypoglycemia and hypoinsulinemia following oral glucose administration. This phenomenon was seen in three patients who survived their disease. Whether the pattern is related to secretion of the hypothalamic hormone somatostatin is unknown.

Abnormal carbohydrate metabolism has also been reported in patients with chondrosarcoma and fibrosarcoma.[11][12] One author has also advanced a hypothesis suggesting that anabolic steroid hormones may promote neoplasia of bone and bone marrow at adolescence.[13]

Familial and Genetic Factors

Incidences of osteosarcoma in siblings have been reported in several families.[14-21] The disease has also been observed in a father and daughter.[19-21] An increasing number of reports have also described an association between retinoblastoma, particularly a bilateral familial type, and the subsequent development of osteosarcoma of the lower extremities.[7][22][23] Two siblings with bilateral retinoblastoma in infancy later developed osteosarcoma of the femur (at 9 and 11 years of age, respectively).[18] Bilateral retinoblastoma is genetically transmitted as an autosomal dominant. The foregoing data suggest that a similar genetic influence may possibly go on to produce osteosarcoma.

Familial tendencies for the development of other forms of bone cancer have also been suggested by a series of reports of siblings affected with Ewing's sarcoma and chondrosarcoma.[24][25] More recently, a new familial cancer syndrome has been suggested by the detection of benign and malignant tumors including retinoblastoma, carcinoma of the bladder, and a possible case of multifocal osteosarcoma.[26] The occurrence of osteosarcoma in one child and other malignant tumors in a brother or sister has also been reported.[14][27][28] The literature further documents several pedigrees with mammary adenocarcinoma, fibrosarcoma, brain tumors, adrenocortical neoplasms, or osteosarcoma.[14][29][30] More rarely, osteosarcoma may arise in an abnormal bone.[31][32]

Ethnic Factors

Several investigators have reported ethnic differences in the incidence of bone cancer. For example, Ewing's sarcoma virtually does not occur in blacks or in the Japanese.[33][34] The very rare incidence of this disease in racial groups native to Africa has also been observed.[35][36] This suggests a form of genetic resistance. In contrast, there is no great difference between the incidence of osteosarcoma in blacks and in whites.

Immune Defects

Persons with primary immune deficiency and cytogenetic syndromes are prone to certain cancers, particularly lymphoma and leukemia.[37] Malignant non-Hodgkin's lymphoma of bone is occasionally encountered in the pediatric age group, and conversion to acute lymphoblastic leukemia in this condition is not unusual. The etiology of the disease, therefore, may be linked to the etiology of leukemia. However, there is no known relationship between the etiology of leukemia and that of other primary bone cancers.

Target Cell

The study of primary tumors of the musculoskeletal system inevitably leads to the conclusion that they represent a continuum of malignant processes originating in the mesenchymal cell. Such tumors exhibit overlapping features, and represent various degrees of differentiation of connective tissue, muscle, smooth muscle, cartilage, and bone. Jeffree and Price have aptly stated that today's fibroblast may be tomorrow's osteoclast.[38]

The interrelationship of bone and soft tissue is evidenced by osteocytic and chondrocytic tumors originating in soft tissues, and by chondrocytic elements in metastatic soft tissue sarcomas such as cystosarcoma phyllodes.[39-43] Osteosarcoma has also been detected in solitary enchondroma, fibrous dysplasia, Maffucci's syndrome, and osteocartilaginous exostosis.[44-49]

ENVIRONMENTAL FACTORS

Viruses

Both soft tissue and skeletal induced oncornavirus sarcomas have been identified in mice, rats, and wooly monkeys.[50 51] However, most of the sarcomagenic viruses of animals are incomplete and require coinfection with leukemia viruses to form the viral genome fragment necessary for synthesis of the viral envelope in the host cells. That this mechanism is responsible for human sarcomas remains to be determined.

In hamsters, the incidence of "spontaneous" osteosarcoma is low. However, osteosarcomas have developed after inoculation with filtrate from human osteosarcoma.[52] Sera from patients with osteosarcoma have also reacted immunologically with these hamster osteosarcomas. This implies that the hamster tumors were induced by human osteosarcoma virus.[53]

In man, antibody and cell-mediated reactions against soft tissue and skeletal sarcomas have also been demonstrated. In particular, studies by Eilber and Morton reveal that antibodies were present in osteosarcoma patients and in 85% of their normal, healthy family members.[54] In contrast, only 29% of normal blood donors showed antibody.

These data would imply a viral etiology, though as yet, there is no concrete evidence that osteosarcoma is caused by a virus or that malignant neoplasms are contagious in the usual sense. Intense, broadly based biologic research is currently in progress, and the demonstration that a virus can be implemented in the etiology of human cancers would not be unexpected.

Trauma

Trauma is usually associated with the discovery of bone tumors, particularly osteosarcoma, and this is generally considered to be coincidental. It is of interest, however, that some bone infarcts have been shown to be present in the development of osteosarcoma in man.[55] Tumors of various types have been observed on the walls of bone cysts and have complicated chronic osteomyelitic sinuses.[56] This has led to the hypothesis that bone disorders with prolonged periods of excessive cellular activity are prone to producing neoplastic change.

Ionizing Radiation

Ionizing radiation is oncogenic in man and has been responsible for the development of leukemia and other human cancers, including osteosarcoma, chondrosarcoma, and fibrosarcoma.[57-59] Radium 224 has been implicated in the development of bone sarcoma in 30 of 270 patients under the age of 20 who were treated empirically for tuberculosis.[60] The sarcoma developed at sites other than those of the primary tuberculous infection. Similar sarcomas have been documented in radium-watch-dial workers and radium chemists.[61 62]

Therapeutically administered external beam irradiation has also been implicated in the development of osteosarcoma. Tumors developed following therapy administered for a variety of benign and malignant conditions. The doses of radiation varied from 800 rad (for bursitis) to 1,300 rad (for retinoblastoma).[63 64] Postirradiation osteosarcomas have also developed in extraosseous tissue following treatment for diseases of the colon, uterine cervix, and base of the brain (suprasellar area, for pituitary tumors).[65-67] Similar factors have been linked to the development of chondrosarcomas.[68 69] No excess of bone cancer has, however, resulted from whole-body irradiation among the atomic bomb survivors in Japan.[70] Furthermore, no correlation has been found between bone cancer mortality in various countries and measurements of radioactivity in drinking water.[71] Thus, ionizing radiation would appear to be associated with development of cancer only through external high-dose irradiation as used in cancer therapy, and through external bone-seeking radioisotopes in occupational or medicinal use.[58 72]

Chemicals

No chemically induced bone tumors have been identified in man, although the risk of chemical carcinogenesis has been demonstrated in laboratory animals. This has been reported with such diverse agents as methylcholanthrene 20, beryllium oxide, and zinc beryllium silicate.[73-77] However, the risk of bone cancer in beryllium workers does not appear to be elevated.[78] Of as yet undertermined significance is the report of development of osteosarcoma in a patient with thalidomide embryopathy.[79]

Studies to determine the etiology of cancer are currently investigating host, epidemiologic, and environmental factors. The immunologic surveillance system is also under examination. Medical knowledge and discoveries gained in these areas will undoubtedly be applied to attempts not only to identif; but also to avoid the causes of human bone cancer. At present, however, despite an increasing volume of literature and anecdotal cases, and an increasing number of research activity, this etiology remains unknown.

REFERENCES

1. *Vital Statistics of the United States, 1973*. Vol. 2, Part B. US Department of Health, Education, and Welfare, Public Health Service, 1975.

2. *Incidence of Childhood Cancer in Harris County, Texas, 1958–1970*, Leukemia Section, Center for Disease Control. February, 1972.

3. Young J.L., Jr. and Miller, R.W.: Incidence of malignant tumors in United States children. *J Pediatr* 86:254–258, 1975.

4. Tjalma, R.A.: Canine bone sarcoma: estimation of relative risks as a function of body size. *J Natl Cancer Inst* 36:1137–1150, 1966.

5. Fraumeni, J.F., Jr.: Stature and malignant tumors of bone in childhood and adolescence. *Cancer* 20:967–973, 1967.

6. Miller, R.W.: Relation between cancer and congenital defects: an epidemiologic evaluation. *J Natl Cancer Inst* 40:1079–1085, 1968.

7. Glass, A.G. and Fraumeni, J.F., Jr.,: Epidemiology of bone cancer in children. *J Natl Cancer Inst* 44:187–199, 1970.

8. Price, C.H.G.: Primary bone-forming tumours and their relationship to skeletal growth. *J Bone Joint Surg* [Br] 40:574–593, 1958.

9. McMaster, J.H.: Carbohydrate metabolism in osteosarcoma. *Orthop* (SICOT) 1:19–21, 1977.

10. Scranton, P.E., Jr., McMaster, J.H., Kenny, F.M. et al: Investigation of carbohydrate metabolism and somatomedin in osteosarcoma patients. *J Surg Oncol* 7:403–409, 1975.

11. Marcove, R.C. and Francis, K.L.: Chondrosarcoma and altered carbohydrate metabolism. *N Engl J Med* 268:1399–1401, 1963.

12. Turner, M. and Horne, C.: Primary fibrosarcoma of lung and diabetes mellitus. *Br J Surg* 57:713–715, 1970.

13. Acheson, R.M.: A hypothesis regarding the possible role of anabolic steroid hormones as promoters of neoplasia of bone and bone marrow at adolescence. *Yale J Biol Med* 36:43–52, 1963.

14. Miller, C.W. and McLaughlin, R.E.: Osteosarcoma in siblings: report of two cases. *J Bone Joint Surg* 59A:261–262, 1977.

15. Harmon, T.P. and Morton, K.S.: Osteogenic sarcoma in four siblings. *J Bone Joint Surg* 48B:493–498, 1966.

16. Pohle, E.A., Stovall, W.D., and Boyer, H.N.: Concurrence of osteogenic sarcoma in two sisters. *Radiology* 27:545–548, 1936.

17. Roberts, C.W. and Roberts, C.P.: Concurrent osteogenic sarcoma in brother and sisters. *JAMA* 105:181–185, 1935.

18. Schimke, R.N., Lowman, J.T., and Cowan, G.A.B.: Retinoblastoma and osteogenic sarcoma in siblings. *Cancer* 34:2077-2079, 1974.

19.Swaney, J.J.: Familial osteogenic sarcoma. *Clin Orthop* 97:64-68, 1973.

20. Epstein, L.I., Bixler, D., and Bennett, J.E.: An incident of familial cancer including three cases of osteogenic sarcoma. *Cancer* 25:889-891, 1970.

21. Mulvihill, J.J., Gralnick, H.R., Whang-Peng, J. et al: Multiple childhood osteosarcomas in an American Indian family with erythroid macrocytosis and skeletal abnormalities. *Cancer* 40:3115-3122, 1977.

22. Jensen, R.D. and Miller, R.W.: Retinoblastoma: epidemiologic characteristics. *N Engl J Med* 285:307-311, 1971.

23. Bolande, R.P.: Childhood tumors and their relationship to birth defects. In Mulvihill, J.J., Miller, R.W., and Fraumeni, J.F., Jr. (eds): *Genetics of Human Cancer.* Raven Press, New York, 1977, pp 43-75.

24. Hutter, R.V.P., Francis, K.C., and Foote, F.W., Jr.: Ewing's sarcoma in siblings: report of the second known occurrence. *Am J Surg* 107:598-603, 1964.

25. Schajowicz, F. and Bessone, J.E.: Chondrosarcoma in three brothers: a pathological and genetic study. *J Bone Joint Surg* 49:129-141, 1967.

26. Chan, H. and Pratt, C.B.: A new familial cancer syndrome? A spectrum of malignant and benign tumors including retinoblastoma, carcinoma of the bladder and other genitourinary tumors, thyroid adenoma, and a probable case of multifocal osteosarcoma. *J Natl Cancer Inst* 58:205-207, 1977.

27. Miller, R.W.: Deaths from childhood leukemia and solid tumors among twins and other siblings in the United States, 1960-67. *J Natl Cancer Inst* 46:203-209, 1971.

28. Draper, G.J., Head, M.M., and Kinnier-Wilson, L.M.: Occurrence of childhood cancers among siblings and estimation of familial risks. *J Med Genet* 19:81-90, 1977.

29. Bottomley, R.H., Trainer, A.L., and Condit, P.T.: Chromosome studies in a 'cancer family.' *Cancer* 28:519-528, 1971.

30. Fraumeni, J.F., Jr., Vogel, C.L., and Easton, J.M.: Sarcomas and multiple polyposis in a kindred. *Arch Intern Med* 121:57-61, 1968.

31. Klenerman, L., Ockenden, B.G., and Townsend, A.C.: Osteosarcoma occurring in osteogenesis imperfecta. *J Bone Joint Surg* 49B:314-323, 1967.

32. Knight, J. and David, S.: Sarcomatous change in three brothers with diaphyseal aclasis. *Br Med J* 1:1013-1015, 1960.

33. Miller, R.W.: Ethnic differences in cancer occurrence: genetic and environmental influences, with particular reference to neuroblastoma. In Mulvihill, J.J., Miller, R.W., Fraumeni, J.F., Jr. (eds): *Genetics of Human Cancer.* New York, Raven Press, 1977, pp 1-4.

34. Jensen, R.D. and Drake, R.M.: Rarity of Ewing's tumour in Negroes. *Lancet* 1:777, 1970.

35. Davies, J.N.P.: Childhood tumours. In Templeton, A.C. (ed): *Tumours in a Tropical Country.* Springer-Verlag, Berlin, 1973, pp 306-343.

36. Williams, A.O.: Tumors of childhood in Ibadan, Nigeria. *Cancer* 36:370-378, 1975.

37. Fraumeni, J.F., Jr.: Genetic factors. In Holland, J.F. and Frei, E., III (eds): *Cancer Medicine.* Lea & Febiger, Philadelphia, 1973, pp 7-15.

38. Jeffree, G.M. and Price, C.H.G.: Bone tumors and their enzymes: a study of the phosphatases, nonspecific esterases and betaglucuronidase of osteogenic and cartilaginous tumours, and fibroblastic and giant cell lesions.

J Bone Joint Surg 47B:120-136, 1965.

39. Wurlitzer, E., Ayala, A., and Romsdahl, M.M.: Extraosseous osteogenic sarcoma. *Arch Surg* 105:691-695, 1972.

40. Stout, A.P. and Verner, E.W.: Chondrosarcoma of the extraskeletal soft tissues. *Cancer* 6:581-590, 1953.

41. Moore, J.P. and Shannon, E.: Extraskeletal chondrosarcoma. *Tex Med* 70:65-68, 1974.

42. Smith, M.T., Farinacci, C.J., Carpenter, H.A. et al: Extraskeletal myxoid chondrosarcoma: a clinicopathological study. *Cancer* 37:821-827, 1976.

43. Fernandez, B.B., Hernandez, F.J., and Spindler, W.: Metastatic cystosarcoma phyllodes: a light and electron microscope study. *Cancer* 37:1737-1746, 1976.

44. Rockwell, M.A. and Enneking, W.H.: Osteosarcoma developing in solitary enchondroma of the tibia. *J Bone Joint Surg* 53A:341-344, 1971.

45. Huvos, A.G., Higinbotham, N.L., and Miller, T.R.: Bone sarcomas arising in fibrous dysplasia. *J Bone Joint Surg* 54A:1047-1056, 1972.

46. Gorlin, R.J. and Sedano, H.: Maffucci's syndrome. *Mod Med* 41:82E, 1973.

47. Braddock, G.T.F. and Hadlow, V.D.: Osteosarcoma in enchondromatosis (Ollier's disease): report of a case. *J Bone Joint Surg* 48B:145-149, 1966.

48. Dahlin, D.C. and Coventry, M.B.: Osteogenic sarcoma: a study of 600 cases. *J Bone Joint Surg* 49A:101-110, 1967.

49. McKenna, R.J., Schwinn, C.P., Soog, K.Y. et al: Sarcomata of the osteogenic series (osteosarcoma, chondrosarcoma, parosteal osteogenic sarcoma, and sarcomata arising in abnormal bone): an analysis of 552 cases. *J Bone Joint Surg* 48A:1-26, 1966.

50. Fujinaga, S., Poel, W.E., and Dmochowski, L.: Light and electron microscope studies of osteosarcomas induced in rats and hamsters by Harvey and Moloney sarcoma viruses. *Cancer Res* 30:1698-1702, 1970.

51. Soehner, R.L. and Dmochowski, L.: Induction of bone tumours in rats and hamsters with murine sarcoma virus, and their cell-free transmission. *Nature* 224:191-193, 1969.

52. Maruyama, K., Dmochowski, L., Romero, J.J. et al: Studies of human cells infected by leukemia viruses. *Bibl Haematol* 39:852-879, 1973.

53. Pritchard, D.J., Reilly, C.A., Finkel, M.P. et al: Cytotoxicity of human osteosarcoma sera to hamster sarcoma cells. *Cancer* 34:1935-1939, 1974.

54. Eilber, F.R. and Morton, D.L.: Sarcoma-specific antigens: detection by complement fixation with serum from sarcoma patients. *J Natl Cancer Inst* 44:651-656, 1970.

55. Dorfman, H.D.: Malignant transformation of benign bone lesions. In *Proceedings*. Seventh National Cancer Conference. J.B. Lippincott Co., Philadelphia, 1973, p 901.

56. Johnston, R.M. and Miles, J.S.: Sarcomas arising from chronic osteomyelitic sinuses: a report of two cases. *J Bone Joint Surg* 55A:162-168, 1973.

57. Ichimaru, M. and Ishimaru, T.: Leukemia and related disorders. *J Radiat Res* 16(suppl):89-96, 1975.

58. Wood, J.W., Tamagaki, H., Nerishi, S. et al: Thyroid carcinoma in atomic bomb survivors, Hiroshima and Nagasaki. *Am J Epidemiol* 89:4-14, 1969.

59. Loutit, J.F.: Malignancy from radium. *Br J Cancer* 24:195-207, 1970.

60. Spiess, H. and Mays, C.W.: Bone cancers induced by ^{224}Ra(ThX) in

children and adults. *Health Phys* 19:713–729, 1970.

61. Aub, J.C., Evans, R.D., Hempelmann, L.H. et al: The late effects of internally deposited radioactive materials in man. *Medicine* 31:221–329, 1952.

62. United Nations: *Report of the United Nations Scientific Committee on the Effects of Atomic Radiation.* General Assembly, Official Records. Nineteenth Session, Supplement no. 14 (A/5814). New York, 1964.

63. Glicksman, A.S. and Toker, C.: Osteogenic sarcoma following radiotherapy for bursitis. *Mt Siani J Med NY* 43:163–167, 1976.

64. Lee, W.R., Laurie, J., and Townsend, A.L.: Fine structure of a radiation-induced osteogenic sarcoma. *Cancer* 76:1414–1425, 1975.

65. Boch, C.: Postirradiation osteogenic sarcoma. *Am J Roentgenol* 87:1157–1162, 1962.

66. Paik, H.H. and Wilkinson, E.J.: Peritoneal osteosarcoma following radiation therapy for ovarian cancer. *Obstet Gynecol* 47:488–491, 1976.

67. Amine, A.R.C. and Sugar, O.: Suprasellar osteogenic sarcoma following irradiation for pituitary adenoma. *J Neurosurg* 44:88–91, 1976.

68. Peimer, C.A., Yuan, H.A., and Sagerman, R.H.: Postirradiation chondrosarcoma. *J Bone Joint Surg.* 58A:1033–1036, 1976.

69. Fitzwater, J.E., Cabaud, H.E., and Farr, G.H.: Radiation-induced chondrosarcoma. *J Bone Joint Surg* 58A:1037–1039, 1976.

70. Yamamoto, T. and Wakabayshi, T.: Bone tumors among the atomic bomb survivors of Hiroshima and Nagasaki. *Acta Pathol Jpn* 19:201–212, 1969.

71. Boyd, J.T., Doll, R., Hill, G.B. et al: Mortality from primary tumours of bone in England and Wales, 1961–63. *Br J Prev Soc Med* 23:12–22, 1969.

72. Sim, F.H., Cupps, R.E., Dahlin, D.C. et al: Postirradiation sarcoma of bone. *J Bone Joint Surg* 54A:1479–1489, 1972.

73. Brunschwig, A.: Production of primary bone tumors (fibrosarcoma of bone) by intramedullary injection of methylcholanthrene. *Am J Cancer* 34:540–542, 1938.

74. Dutra, F.R. and Largent, E.J.: Osteosarcoma induced by beryllium oxide. *Am J Pathol* 26:197–209, 1950.

75. Barnes, J.M., Denz, F.A., and Sissons, H.A.: Beryllium bone sarcomata in rabbits. *Br J Cancer* 4:212–222, 1950.

76. Cloudman, A.M., Vining, D., Barkulis, S. et al: Bone changes observed following intravenous injections of beryllium, abstract ed. *Am J Pathol* 25:810–811, 1949.

77. Gardner, L.U. and Heslington, H.F.: Osteosarcoma from intravenous beryllium compounds in rabbits, abstracted. *Fed Proc* 5:221, 1946.

78. International Agency for Research on Cancer: IARC Monographs on the Evaluation of Carcinogenic Risk of Chemicals to Man. Vol. 1. Lyon, 1972, pp 17–28.

79. Teppo, L., Saxen, E., Tervo, T. et al: Thalidomide-type malformations and subsequent osteosarcoma. *Lancet* 2:405, 1977.

2 Malignant Bone Tumors: Principles and Controversies in Treatment

Norman Jaffe, M.B.Bch., Dip.Paed.

1. Histologic diagnosis
2. Assessment of extent of disease
3. Multidisciplinary approach
4. Discussion with patient and parents
5. Treatment of the primary lesion
   a. Limb preservation
   b. Radiation therapy
6. Adjuvant chemotherapy
7. Treatment of clinically evident metastases
   a. Early metastatic disease
   b. Advanced metastatic disease
8. Palliation
9. Follow-up evaluation

During the past decade, major progress in the diagnosis and treatment of malignant bone tumors has been forged. This may be attributed to advances in clinical and experimental investigation and to contributions from associated disciplines. The results have done much to dispel preexisting tides of pessimism, and they augur an era of cautious optimism.

Advances are usually associated with changing concepts, and this is true in regard to bone tumors, also. This monograph is designed to present the state of the art and to consolidate our knowledge in the management of these tumors. That future changes will occur is undisputed, as, indeed, is the realization that considerable controversy has emerged with the new forms of management. These will be outlined in a discussion of the general principles of treatment.

HISTOLOGIC DIAGNOSIS

Meticulous histologic identification of the tumor is basic to planning an appropriate course of therapy as it assists in differentiating primary malignant tumors of bone and metastatic infiltration from other sources. Those tumors which most frequently metastasize to bone include neuroblastoma, rhabdomyosarcoma, and soft tissue sarcoma. Occasionally, Ewing's sarcoma must be differentiated from non-Hodgkin's lymphoma of bone and early leukemia, and osteosarcoma from fibrosarcoma and chondrosarcoma. Certain malignancies are more responsive to radiation therapy (eg, Ewing's sarcoma and non-Hodgkin's lymphoma of bone), while surgery is the primary mode of therapy for osteosarcoma, chondrosarcoma, fibrosarcoma, and giant cell tumors of bone. The basic tumor type also dictates the nature of the adjuvant chemotherapeutic program to be administered.

ASSESSMENT OF EXTENT OF DISEASE

Following identification of the neoplasm, the full extent of its involvement is determined. Certain tumors characteristically metastasize to particular sites. These must be investigated with currently available techniques. Good-quality radiographs of the entire affected bone are obtained. Occasionally, laminograms may be required to determine the extent of tumor invasion into the medullary cavity or cortex, particularly in parosteal lesions. Local filtration into soft tissue may also be noted.

Most bone tumors metastasize to the lungs. Radiographic examination of the chest, therefore, is a routine procedure. If the chest radiograph is normal, or if only a few metastases are detected, complete lung tomograms should be obtained. Occasionally, chest fluoroscopy may be indicated. Computerized axial tomography is currently under investigation and may prove an additional powerful tool for detecting early pulmonary metastases.

Bone scintigraphy has become a routine procedure of investigation in most centers. This technique may demonstrate abnormalities in bone several months before these would be evident with the conventional radiograph.[1] A positive result calls for radiographic examination of the diseased area. Angiography may be employed to determine the extent of tumor infiltration into adjacent soft tissues, particuarly if limb preservation procedures are being considered.

Biopsies are performed in the operating room, with the patient under general anesthesia and a tourniquet applied to the limb above the tumor. In some centers, needle biopsy is employed. (The importance of biopsy technique is stressed in Chapter 8.) Bone marrow aspirations may be obtained at the same time as the biopsy specimen if spread to other sites is suspected. Prechemotherapy evaluation includes a hemogram, liver function studies, serum electrolytes, blood urea nitrogen and urine analysis. A creatinine clearance study is obtained if methotrexate treatment is to be administered.

MULTIDISCIPLINARY APPROACH

Optimum management of bone tumors can only be achieved through a multidisciplinary approach. The initial diagnosis and assessment of the extent of disease provide an opportunity for the relevant disciplines to integrate and adopt a therapeutic plan of management. When the result of the investigations are available, a conference with the orthopedic surgeon, radiation therapist, and pediatric medical oncologist is scheduled. Preferably, the radiologist, pathologist, social worker, and psychiatrist should also be in attendance. Decisions to amputate are relayed to the prosthetist and physiotherapist, who will provide gait training and also supervise a plan of orthopedic exercises developed by the orthopedist to prevent late contractures in patients undergoing radiation therapy. The social worker and psychiatrist will help the family adjust to changing circumstances.

DISCUSSION WITH PATIENT AND PARENTS

The final diagnosis and projected plan of management are eventually presented to the patient and parents. Representatives from the major disciplines should also be present. If an amputation is contemplated, the patient should be advised that this is being done to remove the tumor. The information should be conveyed several days before the operation to allow the opportunity for the patient to ask questions and to become accustomed to the concept of losing a limb. The reason for the surgery should not be disguised as "infection." This may invoke fear of possible amputation in the patient or his siblings should true infection of a limb subsequently occur.

TREATMENT OF THE PRIMARY LESION

Treatment is designed with curative intent unless the disease is fairly extensive, in which case palliation is the major consideration. The primary tumor is a major determinant of the prognosis since it presents an uninhibited source of metastases. The first objective of treatment, therefore, is to eradicate the primary tumor. This may be accomplished through surgery and/or radiation therapy.

Surgical ablation is usually undertaken for osteosarcoma, fibrosarcoma, and chondrosarcoma. Osteosarcoma is the tumor which has provided the most experience. Two methods of ablation are practiced: disarticulation and transmedullary amputation. (The controversy surrounding the choice of method is discussed in Chapter 8.) Disarticulation removes possible foci of tumor beyond apparently uninvolved marrow. These are referred to as "skip" areas and are not demonstrable by radiographic examination.[2] In contrast, transmedullary amputation has obvious advantages in terms of a functional prosthesis. However, such an approach may be justified only if the cure rate is not affected and is not complicated by tumor recurrence in the stump.

A solution to the controversy is not readily available. The existence of "skip" areas has been discounted in two separate investigations, although the scientific accuracy of the studies has been questioned.[2-4] Further, current radiologic techniques, including bone scanning, may permit more confident planning of a transmedullary amputation, and with effective chemotherapy, residual microscopic disease may be destroyed.

The dilemma surrounding stump recurrence appears more complex. Incidences of from 2% to 16% have been reported.[5-7] However, an accurate assessment is not possible since local recurrence may also be a manifestation of widespread bony metastases.[6] The incidence would be expected to be greater in nonextremity lesions, where radical surgical procedures are not feasible, and when amputation is preceded by repeated attempts at definitive (local) excision.[8] In nonextremity lesions the local recurrence rate may be as high as 85%.[8]

There apparently has been only one study which has attempted to detect differences in survival between the two surgical approaches. This was a retrospective review, and no difference was detected.[3] Despite these results and the accumulating data on absence of local recurrence with treatment with transmedullary amputation and chemotherapy, uniform agreement for its adoption has not been attained.

Limb Preservation

Effective chemotherapy has also achieved reduction in the size of the primary tumor. This has been used as a preoperative measure for limb preservation in several centers while a suitable endoprosthesis is being manufactured. Clinical and pathologic examinations reveal tumor destruction varies from 80% to 100%.[9-11] Central to the decision to recommend limb preservation is the feasibility of performing an adequate cancer operation ab initio. This is determined through clinical and radiographic examinations, bone scintigraphy, and angiography. Factors influencing the decision also include the age of the patient, the size and location of the lesion, and the extent of soft tissue involvement. For lesions of the lower extremities, the patient should have attained full or near full growth. (See Chapters 8, 9, and 10.)

Preoperative treatment with chemotherapy may also provide a powerful hedge against pulmonary micrometastases. The efficacy of such treatment may be gauged by examining the resected specimen: extensive destruction of tumor provides additional support for the use of chemotherapy as adjuvant treatment. Recently, this approach has been adopted for patients undergoing amputation at the Memorial Sloan-Kettering Cancer Center (Chapter 7).

However, controversy surrounds the use of preoperative chemotherapy. Its administration constitutes a delay in initiating surgical treatment, and total tumor destruction is not always achieved. Whether such chemotherapy will still be effective clinically against micrometastases is unknown, although the kinetics of tumor growth suggest that such metastases, unlike large primary tumors, are more sensitive to certain anticancer agents.[12] Until more information is accumulated, however, the Sidney Farber Cancer Institute will continue to carry out limb preservation by immediate resection. Prefabricated endoprostheses have been acquired for this purpose, and preoperative chemotherapy is administered only in exceptional circumstances (Chapter 7).

Radiation Therapy

Radiation therapy is used in treating the primary tumors of Ewing's sarcoma, reticulum cell sarcoma, hemangioendothelial sarcoma, and primary non-Hodgkin's lymphoma of bone (Chapters 13 and 14). Treatment consists of whole-bone irradiation. If there is a lack of response, or if the location of the lesion makes it amenable to surgery, a resection will be performed. In special circumstances, both surgery and radiation therapy will be utilized (as in Ewing's sarcoma of the rib, Chapter 13). This technique is currently also under consideration for high-risk lesions of the pelvis or other areas.*

Concern is occasionally expressed in regard to the ability to achieve permanent local control with radiation therapy. This is of fundamental importance if cure is to be achieved. Published reports would suggest that doses of approximately 5,000 rad or more have

---

*M. Nesbit and G. Rosen : personal communication.

yielded local control in 65% to 95% of patients with Ewing's sarcoma.[13][14] Radiation therapy is usually administered in combination with chemotherapy. The extent to which the latter contributes to the result is difficult to assess since reseeding by distant metastases of a site which has previously been damaged by tumor or irradiation cannot be ascertained.

Treatment combining radiation therapy and chemotherapy must be carefully and judiciously integrated to avoid major morbidity. This may include severe fibrosis, leathering of the skin, and pathologic fractures.[15][16] However, effectively applied, radiation therapy permits retention of a viable, functioning limb, and its benefits probably outweigh the potential side effects and the constant threat of development of a delayed, second neoplasm.[17]

Adjuvant Chemotherapy

Surgery and radiation therapy are limited since they are effective only against localized disease. With most malignant bone tumors, there are disseminated microscopic foci of tumor at the time of presentation. This is not evident clinically. To eradicate these metastases and achieve cure, systemic (adjuvant) chemotherapy is administered after treatment of the primary tumor. The forms of adjuvant treatment for osteosarcoma, Ewing's sarcoma, and non-Hodgkin's lymphoma have been described in the literature.[18-27] In some centers, immunotherapy, transfer factor, or interferon therapy is administered also.[28-30] (See Chapters 6 and 7.)

Adjuvant chemotherapy should be introduced early. This recommendation is based on the observation that tumor destruction by drugs follows a first order of kinetics: a given dose of chemotherapy destroys a constant fraction of cells, not a fixed number.[31][32] Hence, when the tumor burden is small, drugs may be effectively administered within limits tolerated by the host. This avoids the necessity of escalating doses (and attendant side effects) to achieve absolute tumor eradication.

The recommendation for early application of adjuvant chemotherapy also draws support from clinical and experimental investigations. Injection of a single malignant cell ultimately leads to the death of a host animal: the more cells inoculated, the shorter the survival. Thus, the length of survival of animals bearing transplanted tumors is inversely related to the quality of tumor cells which have been inoculated or which survive treatment.[33] The increased sensitivity of micrometastases to chemotherapy, outlined earlier, may also be related to this phenomenon.[12] These principles have been successfully applied to the clinical care of patients. Effective chemotherapy—ideally, applied when the malignant cell burden is at its nadir—produces longer disease-free intervals, impressive increases in survival, and high percentages of cures.[34-39]

Adjuvant chemotherapy is usually given for two years. This period has been prescribed by the observation that, with rare exception, children who are alive and free of disease two years after diagnosis and initiation of treatment attain cure. Periodically, the need for shorter periods of treatment, such as 18 months or less, is given consideration. Investigations to determine the advisability of implementing this practice, particularly if agressive early treatment ("front loading") is employed, are currently in progress. Consequently, periodic changes in chemotherapy programs must be anticipated, particularly after evaluation of study results.

The recommendation to incorporate chemotherapy into the management of bone tumors is conditional and is not made without reservation: it may be prescribed for certain patients cured by amputation or radiation therapy. It also involves recurrent periods of hospitalization and expense, and above all, it may be accompanied by severe morbidity and, occasionally, mortality.[15 25 26 40] However, the prognosis for the majority of patients with bone tumors is extremely bleak. In osteosarcoma, only one of five patients treated by amputation alone is cured. Before the introduction of effective chemotherapy, the overall survival of patients with Ewing's sarcoma was approximately 8%.[41] Clearly, until more promising therapeutic strategies are developed, the potential for substantially improving survival appears to reside only with the addition of effective systemic chemotherapy.

TREATMENT OF CLINICALLY EVIDENT METASTASES

Early Metastatic Disease

In contrast to the rationale underlying the use of adjuvant treatment of microscopic disease, treatment of established metastases involves a coordinated multidisciplinary approach. If the objective is one of "curative intent," the patient must undergo continual reassessment. Treatment strategy depends on the number and sites of the metastases, the feasibility of performing surgery, and the sensitivity of the tumor to chemotherapy and radiation therapy. Effectively applied, the latter disciplines may reduce the necessity for frequent surgical intervention. The approach for patients with osteosarcoma has been discussed in the literature and in Chapters 7 and 15.[42 43]

In Ewing's sarcoma, a number of chemotherapeutic programs

have produced tumor regression,[25] [26] and this has provided compelling support for the use of chemotherapy in patients with metastatic disease. However, improvements have usually been temporary. Additional response may be achieved with radiation therapy. Investigations are currently in progress to determine the efficacy of chemotherapy administered principally to destroy microscopic disease and, it is hoped, areas of bulk disease. Radiation therapy is then administered to the areas of bulk disease in an effort to achieve a more durable response.* Surgical ablation of limited residual disease or of isolated tumors which have failed to respond also may be considered.

Advanced Metastatic Disease

Chemotherapy forms the vanguard of treatment. When administered in an aggressive and systematic manner, destruction of tumor may result in impressive responses and it may be possible to move a patient from a "palliative" category to one of "potential cure." If a satisfactory response is achieved, a decision may be made to ablate the primary lesion if this has not been previously performed. Foci of tumor which fail to respond — or foci of residual disease, if limited — may be removed surgically or treated with a combination of radiation therapy and chemotherapy. After complete regression of tumor has been achieved, further treatment with adjuvant chemotherapy should be administered.[42] [43]

Palliation

This form of treatment constitutes the bulk of clinical practice, since cure is usually not attainable when disease is widespread.[44] The decision to give palliative treatment should be made in agreement with the major disciplines. Analgesics are administered judiciously and without restriction. Radiation therapy is indispensable, and chemotherapy may be extremely helpful. Frequently their application reduces tumor bulk and produces palliation and prolongation of useful life. Surgery also may be utilized. In some instances, cervical chordotomy may be recommended. Occasionally the pain in a swollen, functionless limb is so intense that relief may be possible only through amputation. Some patients may benefit by internal fixation. The family should be fully advised of the goals of treatment, and adequate supportive care should be provided.

---

*N. Jaffe and J.R. Cassady, 1978: investigations in progress.

FOLLOW-UP EVALUATION

Continual observation of patients while they are receiving chemotherapy and after termination of treatment is essential. Radiographic examination of the chest and amputated limb is made at regular intervals. All the resources and expertise of a major center must be marshaled to prevent or treat side effects should these occur. The patient should be followed for the rest of his life in order to detect and treat potential late complications, including second malignant neoplasms. Late relapse many years after discontinuation of treatment remains a constant threat.

SUMMARY

Enthusiasm fostered by the introduction of effective chemotherapy for bone tumors has led to new concepts in treatment. Eradication of the primary tumor remains the major role of surgery and/or radiation therapy. However, adjuvant treatment (usually chemotherapy) is used to destroy microscopic disease. Chemotherapy also potentiates the action of radiation therapy, and in some instances it has the surgical approach to the primary tumor. For optimum results, patients should be offered the benefit of an integrated multidisciplinary approach.

REFERENCES

1. McNeil, B.J., Cassady, J.R., Jaffe, N. et al: Fluorine 18 bone scintigraphy in children with osteosarcoma of Ewing's sarcoma. *Radiology* 109:627–631, 1973.

2. Enneking, W.F. and Kagan, A., 'Skip' metastases in osteosarcoma. *Cancer* 36:2192–2205, 1975.

3. Lewis, R.J. and Lots, M.J.: Medullary extension of osteosarcoma. Implications for rational therapy. *Cancer* 33:371–375, 1974.

4. Upshaw, J.E., McDonald, J.R., and Ghormley, R.K.: Extension of primary neoplasms of bone to bone marrow. *Surg Gynecol Obstet* 89:704–714, 1949.

5. Dahlin, D.C. and Coventry, M.D.: Osteogenic sarcoma: a study of 600 cases. *J Bone Joint Surg* 49A:101–110, 1967.

6. Moore, G.E., Gerner, R.E., and Brugarolas, A.: Osteogenic sarcoma. *Surg Gynecol Obstet* 136:359–366, 1973.

7. Sweetnam, R., Knowelden, J., and Seddon, H.: Bone sarcoma. Treatment by irradiation, amputation, or a combination of the two. *Br Med J* 2:363–367, 1971.

8. McKenna, R.J., Schwinn, C.P., Soong, K.Y. et al: Sarcomata of

the osteogenic series (osteosarcoma, fibrosarcoma, chondrosarcoma, parosteal osteogenic sarcoma, and sarcomata arising in abnormal bone): an analysis of 552 cases. *J Bone Joint Surg* 48A:1-26, 1966.

9. Morton, D.L., Eilber, F.R., Townsend, C.M., Jr. et al: Limb salvage from a multidisciplinary treatment approach for skeletal and soft tissue sarcomas of the extremity. *Ann Surg* 184:268-278, 1976.

10. Jaffe, N., Frei, E., III, Traggis, D., et al: Weekly high-dose methotrexate–citrovorum factor in osteogenic sarcoma: Presurgical treatment of primary tumor and of overt pulmonary metastases. *Cancer* 39:45-50, 1977.

11. Rosen, G., Murphy, M.L., Huvos, A.G., et al: Chemotherapy en bloc resection, and prosthetic bone replacement in the treatment of osteogenic sarcoma. *Cancer* 37:1-11, 1976.

12. Schabel, F.M., Jr.: Concepts for systemic treatment of micrometastases. *Cancer* 35:15-24, 1975.

13. Tefft, M., Chabora, B., and Rosen, G.: Radiation in bone sarcoma. A reevaluation in the era of intensive systemic chemotherapy. *Cancer* 39:806-816, 1977.

14. Perez, C.A., Razek, A., Tefft, M., et al: Analysis of local tumor control in Ewing's sarcoma: preliminary results of a cooperative intergroup study. *Cancer* 40:2864-2873, 1977.

15. Tefft, M., Lattin, P.B., Jereb, B. et al: Acute and late effects on normal tissues following combined chemo- and radiotherapy for childhood rhabdomyosarcoma and Ewing's sarcoma. *Cancer* 37:1201-1213, 1976.

16. Lewis, R.J., Marcove, R.C., and Rosen, G.: Ewing's sarcoma—functional effects of radiation therapy. *J Bone Joint Surg* 59(3):325-331, 1977.

17. Li, F.P., Cassady, J.R., and Jaffe, N.: Risk of second tumors in survivors of childhood cancer. *Cancer* 35:1230-1235, 1975.

18. Jaffe, N., Farber, S., Traggis, D. et al: Favorable response of osteogenic sarcoma to high-dose methotrexate with citrovorum rescue and radiation therapy. *Cancer* 31:1367-1373, 1973.

19. Jaffe, N., Traggis, D., Cassady, J.R. et al: The role of high-dose methotrexate with citrovorum factor 'rescue' in the treatment of osteogenic sarcoma. *Int J Radiat Oncol Biol Phys* 2:261-266, 1977.

20. Rosen, G., Tan, C., Sanmaneechai, A. et al: The rationale for multiple-drug chemotherapy in the treatment of osteogenic sarcoma. *Cancer* 35:936-945, 1975.

21. Pratt, C., Shanks, E., Hustu, O. et al: Adjuvant multiple-drug chemotherapy for osteosarcoma of the extremity. *Cancer* 39:51-57, 1977.

22. Sutow, W.W., Gehan, E.A., Vietti, T.J. et al: Multidrug chemotherapy in primary treatment of osteosarcoma. *J Bone Joint Surg* 58A:629–633, 1976.

23. Cortes, E.P., Holland, J.F., Wang, J.J. et al: Amputation and Adriamycin in primary osteosarcoma. *N Engl J Med* 291:998–1000, 1974.

24. Ochs, J., Freeman, A., and Douglass, H.: Clinical trial of Cis-diamminedichloroplatinum (cis pt II) in osteogenic sarcoma. Proc. AACR/ASCO 18:167. (Abstract No. 665).

25. Jaffe, N., Traggis, D., Sallan, S. et al: Improved outlook for Ewing's sarcoma with combination chemotherapy (vincristine, actinomycin D and cyclophosphamide) and radiation therapy. *Cancer* 38:1925–1930, 1976.

26. Rosen, G., Wollner, N., Tan, C. et al: Disease-free survival in children with Ewing's sarcoma treated with radiation therapy and adjuvant four-drug sequential chemotherapy. *Cancer* 33:384–393, 1974.

27. Jaffe, N., Buell, D., Cassady, J.R. et al: Role of staging in childhood non-Hodgkin's lymphoma. *Cancer Treat Rep* 61:1001–1007, 1977.

28. Marsh, B., Flynn, L., and Enneking, W.: Immunologic aspects of osteosarcoma and their application to therapy. A preliminary report. *J Bone Joint Surg* 54A:1367–1397, 1972.

29. Fudenberg, H.H., Levin, A.S., Spitler, L.E. et al: The therapeutic uses of transfer factor. *Hosp Prac* 9:95–104, 1974.

30. Strander, H., Cantell, K., Carlstrom, G. et al: Clinical and laboratory investigations on man: systemic administration of potent interferon to man. *J Natl Cancer Inst* 51:733–742, 1973.

31. Pittillo, R.F., Schabel, F.M., Jr., Wilcox, W.S. et al: Experimental evaluation of potential anticancer agents. XVI. Basic studies of effects of certain anticancer agents on kinetic behavior of model bacterial cell populations. *Cancer Chemother Rep* 47:1–26, 1965.

32. Wilcox, W.S. The last surviving cancer cell: the chances of killing it. *Cancer Chemother Rep* 50:541–542, 1966.

33. Skipper, H.E., Schabel, F.M., Jr., and Wilcox, W.S.: Experimental evaluation of potential anticancer agents. XIII. On the criteria and kinetics associated with 'curability' of experimental leukemia. *Cancer Chemother Rep* 35:1–111, 1964.

34. Pinkel, D.: Five-year follow-up of 'total therapy' of childhood lymphocytic leukemia. *JAMA* 216:648–652, 1971.

35. Holland, J.F. and Glidewell, O.: Oncologists' reply: survival expectancy in acute lymphocytic leukemia, editorial. *N Engl J Med* 287:769–777, 1972.

36. Farber, S.: Chemotherapy in the treatment of leukemia and Wilms' tumor. *JAMA* 198:826–836, 1966.

37. Jaffe, N., Murray, J., Traggis, D. et al: Multidisciplinary treatment for childhood sarcoma. *Am J Surg* 133:405–413, 1977.

38. Ortega, J.A., Rivard, G.E., Isaac, H. et al: The influence of chemotherapy on the prognosis of rhabdomyosarcoma. *Med Pediatr Oncol* 1:227–234, 1975.

39. Sutow, W.W., Sullivan, M.P., Reid, H.L. et al: Prognosis in childhood rhabdomyosarcoma. *Cancer* 25:1384-1393, 1970.

40. Jaffe, N. and Traggis, D.: Toxicity of high-dose methotrexate (NSC-740) and citrovorum factor (NSC-3590) in osteogenic sarcoma. *Cancer Chemother Rep* 6:31–36, 1975.

41. Falk, S. and Alpert, M.: Five-year survival of patients with Ewing's sarcoma. *Surg Gynecol Obstet* 124:319–324, 1967.

42. Jaffe, N., Traggis, D., Cassady, J.R. et al: Multidisciplinary treatment for micrometastatic osteogenic sarcoma. *Br Med J* 2:1039–1041, 1976.

43. Rosen, G., Huvos, A.G., Mosende, C. et al: Chemotherapy and thoracotomy for metastatic osteogenic sarcoma: a model for adjuvant chemotherapy and the radionale for the timing of thoracic surgery. *Cancer* 41:841–849, 1978.

44. Jaffe, N.: Current concepts in the management of disseminated malignant bone disease in childhood. *Can J Surg* 20:537–539, 1977.

3 Pathology of Benign and Malignant Bone Tumors in Children

Fritz Schajowicz, M.D.

Primary bone tumors, although relatively rare, are more frequent in children and adolescents,[1-10] while metastases occur more commonly in adults. This is one of the reasons few pathologists, except those associated with specialized institutions or registries, have an opportunity to study appreciable numbers of cases with good technical standards of preparation and appropriate clinical information.

The incidence of bone tumors abstracted from material filed at the Latin American Registry of Bone Pathology, which includes cases of all age groups, is comparable to that seen at Children's Hospital in Buenos Aires, which treats most of the neoplasms in children in Argentina (Tables 1 and 2).

The study of bone tumors should be approached from a dynamic standpoint, with the pathologist working in close collaboration with an experienced radiologist and clinician. Whenever possible, comparative pathologic and radiographic studies should be made. This basic practice was recommended by the older, Austrian and German schools of pathology and observed by most modern bone pathologists.

Table 1
Incidence of Benign Bone Tumors, 1954 to 1976

Type of Tumor	No. of Cases
Solitary osteochrondroma	165
Multiple osteochondromatosis	24
Osteoid osteoma	54
Solitary bone cyst	111
Aneurysmal bone cyst	51
Eosinophilic granuloma	83
Nonossifying fibroma (metaphyseal fibrous defect)	91
Chondromyxoid fibroma	11
Epiphysial chondroblastoma	4
Monostotic fibrous dysplasia	19
Polyostotic fibrous dysplasia	8
Albright's disease	2
Total	623
Osteoclastoma	1

NOTE: The statistical data were provided through the kindness of Dr. J.C. Derqui, Jr., Head of the Department of Orthopedic Surgery, Children's Hospital, Buenos Aires.

Table 2
Incidence of Malignant Bone Tumors, 1954 to 1976

Type of Tumor	No. of Cases
Osteosarcoma	54
Ewing's sarcoma	49
Chondrosarcoma	2
Justacortical osteosarcoma	1
Juxtacortical chondrosarcoma	1
Fibrosarcoma	2
Osteoblastoma	1
Total	111

NOTE: Statistics compiled by the Department of Orthopedic Surgery, Children's Hospital, Buenos Aires.

In this chapter only the most common bone neoplasms which occur in children, such as osteosarcoma and Ewing's sarcoma, will be discussed in detail. Less attention will be devoted to malignant tumors which are seen only rarely. However, a certain number of benign tumors and several tumorlike lesions which occur in children with reasonable frequency will be discussed since many of these may simulate malignant tumors and lead to inappropriate therapy.

DIAGNOSIS

Radiographic examination is essential to a definitive diagnosis. If necessary, tomography, angiography, and/or bone scan should be employed in addition to routine x-ray examination. Histologic study is essential to a precise diagnosis, and a biopsy is done prior to initiation of surgical, radiation, or chemotherapeutic treatment.

Open surgical biopsy (by incision or excision) is employed in most major centers in the United States, the United Kingdom, and Europe. Elsewhere, aspiration, or trocar, biopsy is used. In all instances, it is most important for the pathologist to be familiar with the clinical and radiologic findings, and he should know the exact origin of the material submitted for analysis.

There is little danger of increased growth or spread of tumor resulting from the biopsy procedure if it is performed competently. Frozen-section diagnosis immediately prior to surgical treatment is utilized by some investigators.[3] However, few pathologists have sufficient experience with such frozen sections to render an immediate, accurate opinion. Also, the approach has failed to improve survival in patients with osteosarcoma, for whom it has principally been employed. Accordingly, treatment decisions are usually deferred until the results of analysis of sections from paraffin-embedded material are available.

At our institution, aspiration (needle) biopsy is used, particularly for lesions where the anatomic site or the proposed treatment makes open biopsy difficult or undesirable.[11-13] Experience in over 8,000 cases, including approximately 2,000 cases with needle biopsies of the spine, has shown the method to be reasonably safe, yielding positive results in over 75% of cases performed in experienced hands and under x-ray control.[11] [12] [13] For vertebral lesions, a special technique described by Valls, Ottolenghi, and Schajowicz has been utilized.[14] With this method, sufficient material for smears and paraffin sections may be obtained, and in some cases bacteriologic examination has also been performed.[12] [13]

The value and/or limitations of histochemical procedures and electron microscopy in the diagnosis of bone tumors will be discussed in the chapters dealing with the relevant tumor types.[15] [16]

CLASSIFICATION

Confusion regarding the nomenclature and classification of bone tumors is fairly widespread. This is largely due to our lack of knowledge of the histogenesis of bone tissue in both normal and pathologic conditions. An ideal classification would be one based on histogenetic or embryogenic concepts, but this goal has not yet been attained. The World Health Organization (WHO), has attempted to establish a universally acceptable classification, based upon morphohistologic criteria, which would be practical and useful to all cancer workers.[8] It involves defining characteristics of tumor cell differentiation and the recognizable types of intercellular material that they produce.[10] This nomenclature, outlined below, permits useful prediction of the properties and behavior of the different tumor types, and it has been adopted for use in this chapter.

LIST

Histologic typing of primary bone tumors and tumorlike lesions*

   I. Bone-Forming Tumors
      A. Benign
         1. Osteoma
         2. Osteoid osteoma and osteoblastoma
            (benign osteoblastoma)
      B. Malignant
         1. Osteosarcoma (osteogenic sarcoma)
         2. Juxtacortical osteosarcoma
            (parosteal osteosarcoma)

  II. Cartilage-Forming Tumors
      A. Benign
         1. Chondroma
         2. Osteochondroma
            (osteocartilaginous exostosis)
         3. Chondroblastoma (benign chondro-
            blastoma, epiphyseal chondroblastoma)
         4. Chondromyxoid fibroma
      B. Malignant
         1. Chondrosarcoma
         2. Juxtacortical chondrosarcoma
         3. Mesenchymal chondrosarcoma

 III. Giant-Cell Tumor (Osteoclastoma)

 IV. Marrow Tumors
         1. Ewing's sarcoma
         2. Reticulosarcoma of bone
         3. Lymphosarcoma of bone
         4. Myeloma

  V. Vascular Tumors
      A. Benign
         1. Hemangioma
         2. Lymphangioma
         3. Glomus tumor (glomangioma)
      B. Intermediate or Indeterminate
         1. Hemangioendothelioma
         2. Hemangiopericytoma

      C. Malignant
         1. Angiosarcoma

VI. Other Connective Tissue Tumors
   A. Benign
      1. Desmoplastic fibroma
      2. Lipoma
   B. Malignant
      1. Fibrosarcoma
      2. Liposarcoma
      3. Malignant mesenchymoma
      4. Undifferentiated sarcoma

VII. Other Tumors
      1. Chordoma
      2. "Adamantinoma" of long bones
      3. Neurilemmoma
         (schwannoma, neurinoma)
      4. Neurofibroma

VIII. Unclassified Tumors

IX. Tumorlike Lesions
      1. Solitary bone cyst
         (simple or unicameral bone cyst)
      2. Aneurysmal bone cyst
      3. Juxta-articular bone cyst
         (intraosseous ganglion)
      4. Metaphyseal fibrous defect
         (nonossifying fibroma)
      5. Eosinophilic granuloma
      6. Fibrous dysplasia
      7. "Myositis ossificans"
      8. "Brown tumor" of hyperparathyroidism

---

*WHO International Reference Center for the Histological Definition and Classification of Bone Tumors and the Latin-American Registry of Bone Pathology.

BONE-FORMING TUMORS

Benign Tumors

Since Jaffe's classic report, the denomination *osteoid osteoma* for a peculiar, rather common benign osteoblastic lesion probably of neoplastic nature, has become universally accepted and familiar to orthopedic surgeons and pathologists.[17] The lesion is characterized by a small core, or nidus, of cellular, highly vascularized tissue made up of a network of trabeculae of immature bone and osteoid tissue in varying proportions (Figure 1). This is surrounded by a conspicuous region of sclerotic bone, the perifocal reactive zone, especially when the lesion develops in or near a cortical portion. According to Jaffe, the nidus tends not to exceed 1.0 cm in diameter, but it may be as large as 2.0 cm in exceptional cases. In addition, the reactive perifocal zone is much more striking when the osteoid osteoma is oriented toward the cortex rather than when it is localized within the spongiosa. In this latter case, there is generally little perifocal sclerosis; in fact, there may be none.

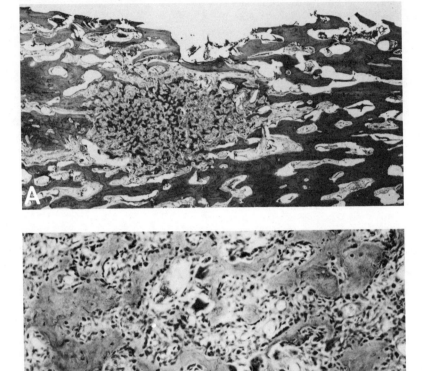

Figure 1 Osteoid osteoma (circumscribed osteoblastoma). Photomicrographs at low (A) and high (B) magnification. (A) Typical central nidus surrounded by sclerotic bone (x 200). (B) Active neoformation of osteoid and incompletely calcified immature bone trabeculae. These are surrounded by rows of osteoblasts alternating with giant cells of osteoclast type and separated by connective tissue rich in hyperemic capillary vessels (x 400).

In contrast to the above, *benign osteoblastoma* is the name proposed independently by Jaffe and by Lichtenstein to designate a rather vascular osteoid and bone-forming benign tumor.[18-20] It is characterized by the abundant presence of osteoblasts, a larger size (usually greater than 1.0 cm in diameter), and the usual absence of any surrounding zone of reactive bone formation. The same lesion had been designated by Dahlin and Johnson as *giant osteoid osteoma* in an attempt to emphasize its close histologic resemblance to osteoid osteoma while at the same time indicating a difference in size to the average tumor.[21] However, in a later publication Dahlin favored the more widely accepted denomination benign osteoblastoma.[3]

According to our observations, osteoid osteoma and osteoblastoma have to be considered as closely related processes of osteoblastic derivation, and it must be emphasized that there are no specific histologic criteria that can be used to distinguish between them.[22] [23] Although some clinical and radiologic differences exist between the smaller osteoid osteoma and the larger osteoblastoma, these differences are, in our opinion, probably the consequence of their locations (cortical and medullary, respectively), as this would explain the slow growth potential of the osteoid osteoma. We have proposed to designate the latter *circumscribed osteoblastoma,* in view of its less active growth relative to benign osteoblastoma. For these reasons, the lesions are reported in the WHO classification under a common heading. The term osteoid osteoma has been retained because of its familiarity and general acceptance, although the denomination osteoblastoma for both entities would be more appropriate.

De Souza Dias and Frost accept our criteria and use the terms *cortical osteoblastoma* for osteoid osteoma and *spongious osteoblastoma* for genuine osteoblastoma.[24]

Osteoid Osteoma is a rather common benign lesion which occurs most frequently in the shaft of long bones, particularly the tibia and femur. It usually occurs during the second decade of life and is more common in males. The lesions are generally painful and relief may be obtained with aspirin.

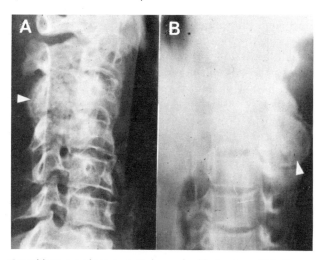

Figure 2   Osteoblastoma of spine. A. Radiograph of lesion (arrow). B. Tomograph of lesion (arrow) affecting apophysis of the third cervical vertebra in a 14-year-old boy. The osteoblastoma is central (medullary) and shows spotty calcification.

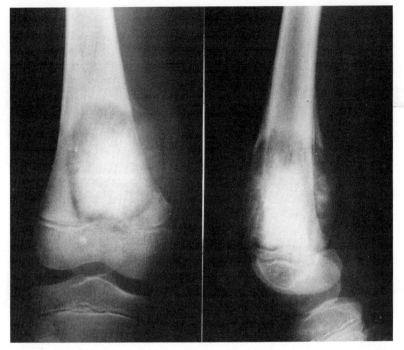

Figure 3 Anteroposterior and lateral radiographs showing osteosarcoma of the lower metaphysis of the femur in a girl 8 years of age. There is predominance of bone sclerosis and a typical Codman's triangle at its upper end.

Osteoblastoma has a histologic structure similar to that of osteoid osteoma, but it occurs less frequently.[3] It primarily affects the short and flat bones, especially the vertebrae, and usually appears during the second and third decades of life. In some cases of higher cellularity and growth activity, histologic distinction from low-grade osteosarcoma may be difficult. Schajowicz and Lemos have described a distinct tumor type—*malignant osteoblastoma* —which they consider the malignant counterpart of osteoblastoma.[25] This process is more common in young adults and differs from conventional osteosarcoma in its clinical features and better prognosis.

Malignant Tumors

Osteosarcoma is the term preferred by WHO and by ourselves to the still widely used *osteogenic sarcoma*. The tumor is characterized by the direct formation of bone or osteoid tissue by the tumor cells (Figure 4). Osteosarcoma is the most common of the primary malignant bone tumors and the one most often seen in children. Of 330 cases filed at the Latin American Registry, its incidence was almost twice that of Ewing's sarcoma or chondrosarcoma. The tumor occurs slightly more often in males and is most commonly encountered in the second decade of life. It is relatively rare below the age of 10, and its incidence is exceptional in individuals under 5 or over 40. Our youngest patient was 2 years old, and some isolated observations of congenital osteosarcoma can be found in the literature. Most tumors developing after middle age are associated with Paget's disease or, more rarely, are secondary to irradiation or fibrous dysplasia.[26-28]

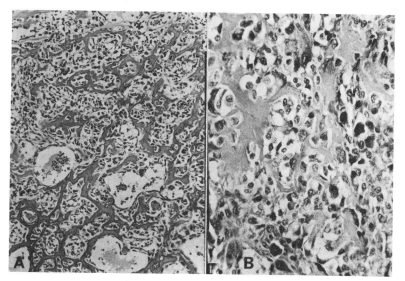

Figure 4 Osteosarcoma. Photomicrographs at low (A, x 100) and higher (B, x 400) magnification show tumor bone and osteoid formation and the conspicuous atypism of the osteoblasts.

Osteosarcoma has a predilection for the metaphyseal area of the long bones: the lower end of the femur (163 of our cases); the upper end of the tibia (62 cases); and, less frequently, the humerus (33 cases). These sites are close to the most active, growing epiphysis. Much less frequent is involvement of the upper metaphysis of the femur (5 cases), the inferior metaphysis of the tibia (7 cases), and the metaphysis or diaphysis of the fibula (15 cases). The diaphysis of other long bones, and also short and flat bones, is rarely involved, among them more commonly the iliac bone (14 cases).

The conventional osteosarcoma, in contrast to the juxtacortical type, arises centrally and, after destroying the cortex, invades the surrounding soft tissues, but it generally respects the adjacent growth cartilage. On gross and radiographic examination, an almost purely osteolytic and sclerosing variety may be distinguished; however, the mixed type is seen more often. The osteolytic variety may simulate a non-bone-forming malignant tumor such as giant cell tumor or fibrosarcoma, or even a benign lesion such as an aneurysmal bone cyst.

An undifferentiated multipotential tumor cell undergoes various stages of differentiation during its skeletal evolution. Accordingly, osteosarcoma shows considerable diverseness in its gross and histologic pattern, varying greatly in the amount of tumor and osteoid present. The tissues of the tumor exhibit pleomorphism, a great number of atypical mitoses, and wide areas of necrosis, but reactive bone formation may be very scarce or totally lacking. This is characteristic of the osteolytic, rapidly growing lesions and may be more or less extensive in the mixed or sclerotic types, giving origin to the characteristic, but not pathognomonic, periosteal reactions of Codman's spur or triangle, and the classical sun-ray pattern (Figures 3 and 5). In addition to bone and osteoid, the tumor cells may produce cartilage and myxoid or fibrous tissue, and many areas may have an undifferentiated spindle-cell pattern without any production of a specific intercellular substance.

Irrespective of the intercellular substances, the primary formation of bone by sarcomatous cells, that is, tumor bone, classifies the

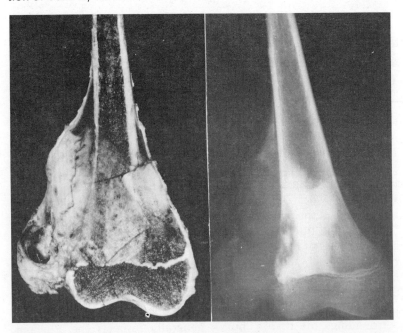

Figure 5 Photograph and radiograph of an osteosarcoma showing the Codman triangle and detention of the tumor at the cartilage growth plate.

tumor as osteosarcoma. In addition, particularly in some rapidly growing, almost purely osteolytic tumors, abundant cavernous vessels or blood-filled spaces may be observed, intermingled with a great number of multinucleated giant cells of osteoclast or tumoral type. This has been designated the "telangiectatic type" of osteosarcoma, and it may be confused with a malignant giant cell tumor or aneurysmal bone cyst (Figure 6).[26] [29] [30]

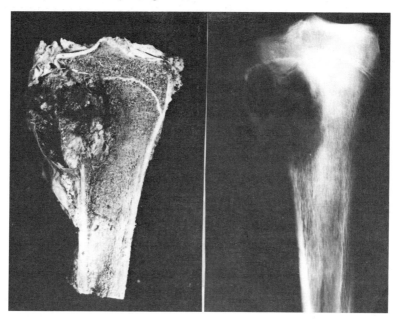

Figure 6 Photograph and radiograph of a gross specimen of an osteosarcoma, telangiectatic type, showing the hemorrhagic and osteolytic pattern of the tumor.

Except perhaps for the telangiectatic variety, which seems to have a worse prognosis, defining subdivisions of osteosarcoma on the basis of predominantly osteoblastic, chondroblastic, or fibroblastic structures (as reported by Dahlin—although also considered academic by him), or according to a variety of gross patterns, does not seem to be useful as far as prognosis is concerned.[26]

It is essential to distinguish tumor bone formation from common, reactive bone formation. Sometimes enchondral ossification, or spicules of calcified cartilage in cartilaginous tumors, may be confused with this appearance. This distinction is often rather difficult, and it accounts for some of the occasions when a cartilage tumor, which generally has a better prognosis, is classified as osteosarcoma.

The histochemical demonstration of alkaline phosphatase, even in apparently undifferentiated tumor cells, may occasionally assist in the identification of osteoblasts which are strongly positive.[11][15] Simultaneously, it may be possible to distinguish tumor bone or osteoid from areas of hyaline fibrous tissue or cartilage.

In metastasis in the majority of patients, the tumor propagates through the blood vessels to the lungs and pleura. These target organs are involved at an early stage. Only rarely are metastases detected in regional lymph glands or other bones or internal organs, except in the final stages of the disease. Bone metastasis has to be distinguished from the rare cases of multifocal osteosarcoma, in which the different lesions, generally of the sclerotic type, appear almost simultaneously, with a symmetrical and bilateral distribution.[31]

Juxtacortical osteosarcoma is the term preferred for a distinctive bone-forming tumor of slow evolution which develops from the surface of a bone—specifically, from the periosteum and immediate parosteal connective tissue. The lesion has been classified by Geschickter and Copeland as *parosteal osteoma,* even though these authors realize its malignant potentialities.[32] Jaffe has classified it as *juxtacortical osteogenic sarcoma;* and Dwinnel, Dahlin, and Ghormley, as *parosteal osteogenic sarcoma.*[5][33] Most tumors show a rather high degree of structural differentiation, which coincides with a better prognosis than for conventional osteosarcoma. It can be mistaken for a benign lesion, particularly myocitis ossificans, if the pathologist is not familiar with the radiologic and histologic features and does not consider the cytologic details of the spindle cell stroma between the generally mature and innocent bony trabeculae.

Juxtacortical osteosarcoma is much less common than central osteosarcoma. We have only 45 cases in our files. The preferred location is the lower end of the femur (22 cases), especially the popliteal region; the upper end of the humerus (8 cases); and less frequently, the tibia (4 cases), fibula (3 cases), and upper femur (3 cases). The tumor is unusual in children, occurring most commonly in those 20 to 40 years old and therefore it will not be discussed in greater detail.[27][34]

CARTILAGE-FORMING TUMORS

With the exception of osteochondroma (osteocartilaginous exostosis), chondroblastoma, and chondromyxoid fibroma, cartilage-forming tumors (benign and malignant) are uncommon in children. For this reason, in this section and in the section dealing with giant cell lesions of bone we will describe only these particular entities in detail.

Benign

Chondroma is a common benign tumor which occurs more frequently in adults. It usually occurs as a single lesion (enchondroma) situated centrally in the tubular bones of the hands and feet, and less frequently in the large limb bones, the ribs, or the flat bones. On rare occasions, chondroma is located peripherally, adjacent to the surface of the bone; it is then designated periosteal, or juxtacortical, chondroma. Infrequently, chondroma may affect several or many bones, especially those of the hand (multiple enchondromatosis). Lesions with widespread involvement and a predominantly unilateral location constitute a developmental defect called Ollier's disease, or dyschondroplasia, or, when accompanied by multiple hemangiomas of soft parts, Maffucci's syndrome.[35-37]

The histologic distinction between chondroma and chondrosarcoma may be difficult, particularly when only limited material is available. Malignant change occurs rarely in solitary enchondroma, especially in those tumors located in hands and feet. But malignant change is frequent, occurring in approximately 25% of cases, in multiple enchondromatosis, with or without Ollier's disease.

Osteochondroma, or osteocartilaginous exostosis, is the most common cartilage lesion and the most frequent benign "tumor" in children. Growth of the lesions usually ceases at the time of skeletal maturation. Consequently, many consider them disorders of growth rather than true neoplasias.

Osteochondroma is characterized by a cartilage-capped bony projection on the external surface of a bone, with either a broad or a narrow base (ie, sessile or pedunculated) arising in the metaphyseal area of, usually, a long, tubular bone. The preferred sites are the lower end of the femur and the upper ends of the humerus and tibia, but not infrequently the scapula or iliac bones (among others) may also be involved.

Osteochondroma is more commonly solitary, but it may be part of a generalized process called multiple hereditary exostosis (hereditary deforming chondrodysplasia, or diaphyseal aclasia).[38 39] Malignant transformation into a secondary chondrosarcoma (peripheral chondrosarcoma) is very rare in solitary osteochondroma, but it occurs in 5% to 7% of cases of multiple exostosis.

Chondroblastoma We have recently reviewed our experiences in epiphyseal chondroblastoma.[40] This is the term we proposed in 1947 for the relatively rare tumor designated *benign chondroblastoma* of bone by Jaffe and Lichtenstein in 1942 and formerly classified as an *epiphyseal chondromatous giant cell tumor*

36

by Codman.[41][42] This distinctive neoplasm usually occurs during the teen years, although occasional cases in older individuals may be observed. The latter seem to be cases with a long evolution which possibly commenced during adolescence and remained stationary or symptomless for many years. The tumor is more common in males (2:1) and most often involves the epiphysis (primary or accessory) of long or short bones adjacent to the epiphyseal cartilage plate (Figure 7), but occasionally it may extend into the adjacent metaphyseal region. Origin in metaphyseal location seems to be exceptional, and only 8 cases have been reported in the literature.[43] The preferred locations, in descending order, are upper end of the tibia, lower and upper end of the femur, and upper end of the humerus.

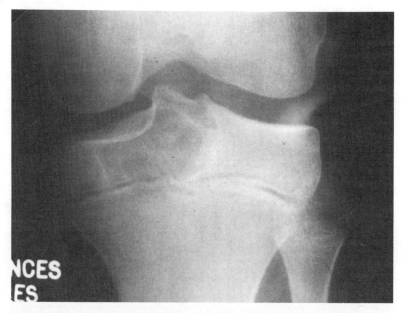

Figure 7   Chondroblastoma of the upper tibial epiphysis in a 12-year-old boy.

Histologically, chondroblastoma is characterized by highly cellular tissue composed of rounded or polygonal cells with fairly distinct cell borders. In our opinion, there are most probably reticulohistiocytic elements possibly originating from cellular structures at the epiphyseal side of the growth cartilage and possessing a definite potential and tendency to develop into poorly differentiated chondroblastic tissue and then into more mature cartilage. These reticulohistiocytic cells may correspond to the structures designated "germ cells" by Jaffe and may be identical to "resting or reserve cells" normally situated at this area of the growth cartilage.[5] The mononuclear tumor cells are always intermingled with a variable number of multinucleated giant cells of the osteoclast type, arranged either singly or in groups (Figure 8). Usually the tumor cells are packed closely together, but in several areas a certain amount of cartilaginous intercellular matrix may be present, showing zones of necrosis and focal calcification which may be visible in the radiographs.

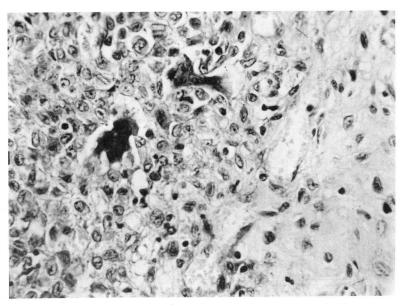

Figure 8 Chondroblastoma. Photomicrograph showing the stromal cells in chondroblastic evalution and some scattered multinucleated giant cells of osteoclast type (x 400).

Approximately 15% of chondroblastomas demonstrate features similar to aneurysmal bone cysts. We have designated these lesions cystic chondroblastomas. Tumors with transitional stages between chondroblastoma and chondromyxoid fibroma also have been observed and make the exact classification of these lesions difficult.[44][45] Occasionally recurrence after curettage may occur, but malignant evolution is very rare and has been reported in only a few cases.[45-49]

Chondromyxoid fibroma is the least common benign cartilaginous tumor. It was described as a distinct entity by Jaffe and Lichtenstein in 1948 and had formerly been classified as a myxoma by Bloodgood, and as a myxomatous variant of the giant cell tumor by Ewing.[50][51] It had also been mistaken for malignant tumors, especially chondrosarcoma and myxosarcoma.

Our experience confirms its predilection for the first two decades, 68% of cases occur in patients between 5 and 25 years of age. In contrast to chondroblastoma, in which males predominate, there is no sex predominance. The most frequent location, in our experience and reported by others, is in the metaphyseal region of a long bone, particularly the upper tibia, followed by other long bones (femur, fibula, and foot) and the tarsal bones.[52] Radiologically, the lesions appear as eccentric, radiolucent areas with slightly sclerotic borders towards the spongiosa which often cause expansion of the thinned cortex (Figure 9).

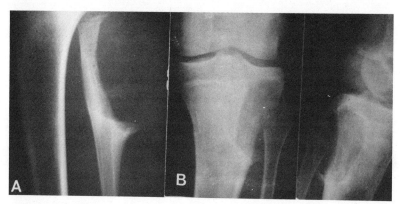

Figure 9 (A) Chondromyxoid fibroma of the upper end of the fibula. Radiograph shows an eccentric expanding lesion well-limited towards the spongiosa. Although the radiographic appearance may cause it to be mistaken for an aneurysmal bone cyst, the macroscopic solid pattern refutes this diagnosis. (B) Chondromyxoid fibroma of the upper metaphysis of the tibia showing the eccentric location and the slightly sclerotic inner borders.

Histologically, the tumor is characterized by lobulated areas of spindle-shaped or stellate cells with abundant myxoid or chondroid intercellular material. These are separated by bands of cellular connective tissue which are rich in spindle-shaped or round cells and are intermingled with a varying number of multinucleated giant cells of the osteoclast type (Figure 10). Cells with nuclear atypism and appearing hyperchromatic, sometimes with globulous or monstrous nuclei, may be present in the myxoid areas. These cells can result in confusion with chondrosarcoma, but they are without sinister implications.

As already mentioned, intermediate, or transitional stages with chondroblastoma do exist. A true myxoma seems to be peculiar to the jaws and apparently has no counterpart, or at least is exceptional, in other bones of the skeleton.[53] The designation of the tumor as a fibroma appears illogical in view of the general agreement that it belongs to the group of cartilage tumors, and in our opinion, the term *fibromyxoid chondroma* would be a more appropriate denomination.

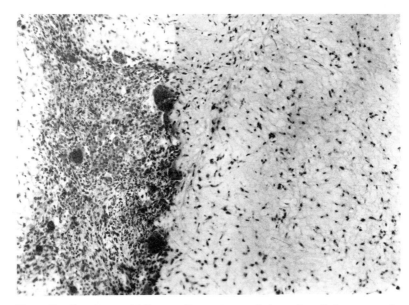

Figure 10 Chondromyxoid fibroma. Photomicrograph shows the cellular aspects of a septum containing multinucleated giant cells (x 100).

Excision or block resection is preferred to curettage as a method of treatment because of the relatively high incidence of recurrence after curettage. However, malignant change seems to be extremely rare.

Malignant Tumors

Chondrosarcoma, which is characterized by formation of atypical cartilage (not bone) by tumor cells, is a relatively common tumor usually seen in adults between 30 and 60 years of age.[54] It is definitely rare in persons under 20 year of age. In the files of the Children's Hospital and the Latin American Registry, only a few cases in children under 15 years of age have been documented.

Chondrosarcoma shows wide variations in its histologic features and behavior, and it is necessary to distinguish between the relatively well differentiated tumors of low-grade malignancy and the more malignant, rapidly growing anaplastic and pleomorphic varieties. Some chondrosarcomas show relatively undifferentiated spindle cell tissue, which probably represents a transformation to highly malignant fibrosarcoma rather than a "dedifferentiation" of a previously well differentiated chondrosarcoma.[55]

Most of the rare chondrosarcomas in children are rapidly growing and highly malignant and should not be misdiagnosed as osteosarcomas, especially of the chondroblastic type. Extensive areas of atypical chondroid formation in chondroblastic osteosarcoma may lead to this error, particularly if only small fragments of the periphery of the tumor are available to the pathologist and the clinical and radiologic features have not been furnished.

Juxtacortical chondrosarcoma is a rare malignant tumor arising from the surface of a long bone. It may be of periosteal origin and has to be distinguished from secondary chondrosarcomatous change in osteochondroma. Juxtacortical chondrosarcoma is possibly the malignant counterpart of juxtacortical osteosarcoma, and as such it definitely has a better prognosis than the conventional central chondrosarcoma of a similar histologic grade. This has been shown in a recent report of nine cases, the majority of which were treated with wide resection and long-term follow-up. Most of the patients were between 10 and 20 years of age.[56]

Mesenchymal chondrosarcoma is a rare tumor and seems to be uncommon in children, but it has sufficient histologic features to permit its definition as a distinct malignant cartilage-forming neoplasm. It is characterized by highly cellular areas containing round cells of an undifferentiated (mesenchymal) variety which resemble Ewing's sarcoma or reticulosarcoma, and by scattered areas of more or less differentiated cartilage. The round cells often show an evident relationship to thin-walled or capillary vessels, resulting in a pattern very similar to hemangiopericytoma.[57]

Nearly one-third of the cases reported and observed by us were of extraosseous origin. We have not discarded the possibility that the tumor represents a mixed mesenchymal growth (malignant mesenchymoma) with a vascular and a cartilaginous component.

MARROW TUMORS

There are no benign tumors in this group. Ewing's sarcoma is the most common malignant neoplasm, and it is the most common tumor in children after osteosarcoma. Primary malignant lymphomas (reticulum cell sarcoma and lymphosarcoma) are very rare under 15 years of age, and multiple myeloma is a tumor which occurs only infrequently in children.

Ewing's Sarcoma

The nature and histogenesis of this tumor have been disputed ever since Ewing described it as "diffuse endothelioma of bone," or "endothelial myeloma," thus defining it as an entity distinct from osteosarcoma, although its derivation from undifferentiated mesenchymal cells of the bone marrow seems highly probable.[58][59] The difficulties of differential diagnosis within the group of malignant round cell tumors of the bone marrow, and specifically of separation between Ewing's sarcoma, malignant lymphoma and metastatic neuroblastoma (sympathoblastoma), are well known.

The preferred locations of Ewing's sarcoma are the metadiaphyseal regions of long bones (femur, tibia, humerus, and fibula), although some flat or short bones, especially the pelvis and scapula, may also be involved. The predominant age is between 5 and 15 years; it is exceedingly rare after the third decade, and uncommon before the fifth year. Males are affected slightly more frequently than females.

The radiologic appearances include a destructive bone lesion, usually accompanied by reactive bone formation, occasionally with the pattern of an "onion skin" periosteal bone formation (Figure 11). The latter, a characteristic but not necessarily diagnostic finding in long bones, is not always found. The typical pattern is absent in flat or short bones. Some benign lesions, especially eosinophilic granuloma or osteomyelitis located in long bones, may simulate the radiographic appearance of Ewing's sarcoma.

Although certain cases may be distinguished from primary reticulum cell sarcoma by clinical and roentgenographic examination, a definite diagnosis must always await histopathologic findings. Proper differentiation between the two entities is imperative because of the vastly better prognosis for reticulum cell sarcoma.

Ewing's sarcoma metastasizes early to the lungs and to other bones.[58] [60] Its striking tendency to involve other bones suggests a multicentric origin. In our experience, metastasis to regional lymph nodes or to the central nervous system is rare. There are, however, a few investigators who do not accept Ewing's sarcoma as a specific entity and who agree with the view expressed by Willis that most cases represent metastasis from neuroblastoma to bone.[61]

In most tumors a medullary origin is evident, although in some cases a cortical or subperiosteal origin with secondary penetration into the marrow cavity may be suspected. Generally, a diffuse infiltration of the bone marrow, with destruction of the spongiosa and invasion of haversian spaces of the cortex, is observed. Involvement of subperiosteal areas with reactive periosteal bone of "onion skin" appearance may also occur. In more advanced cases, extensive destruction of the cortex and invasion of the extraperiosteal region by the tumor may be seen. In a few cases, radial reactive bone spicules are produced. The tumor tissue is generally of a grayish white color and shows hemorrhagic areas; frequently, yellowish zones of extensive necrosis, and an appearance suggesting suppuration, may lead to an erroneous impression of osteomyelitis. Infiltration of the marrow space at a distance greater than is apparent from the radiographic findings may occur. This explains the necessity for irradiating the whole bone.

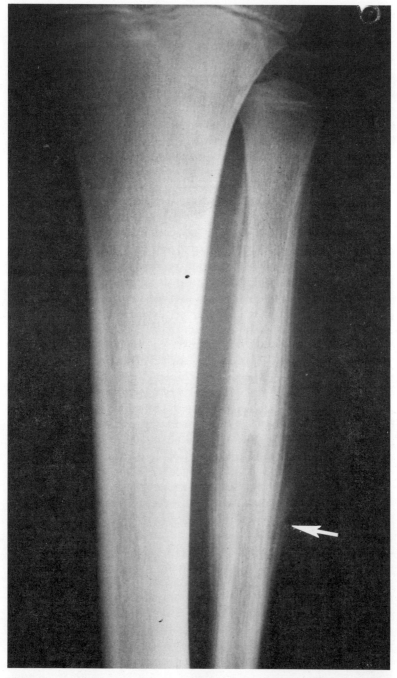

Figure 11 Ewing's sarcoma of the upper third of the fibular shaft in a 13-year-old boy which shows the typical "onion skin" periosteal reactive bone formation (arrow).

Histologically the tumor is characterized by a rather uniform appearance of densely packed cells with round nuclei about two or three times the size of a lymphocyte nucleus (but without distinct cytoplasmic outlines or prominent nucleoli) and by the absence of bone or cartilage formation (Figure 12A). The tumor is divided into irregular strands or lobules by conspicuous septa of fibrous tissue. Mitoses are present but not numerous. Hemorrhages and extensive areas of necrosis are common and occasionally create an apparent perithelial arrangement of viable cells as the necrosis occurs at some distance from the blood vessels. In the zones of necrobiosis, the nuclei are often small and pyknotic, about the size of a lymphocyte. These fields are particularly prone to be mistaken for malignant lymphoma of the lymphocytic type (lymphosarcoma). At times the tumor cells surround small necrotic foci, yielding alveolarlike formations which resemble the rosettes of neuroblastoma.

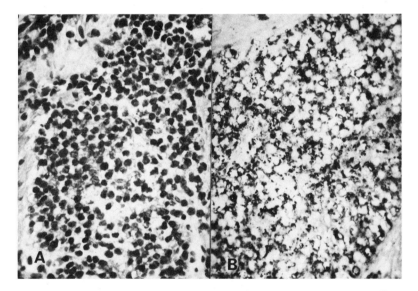

Figure 12 (A) Photomicrograph showing uniform appearance of the tumor cells in Ewing's sarcoma, with regular round nuclei and indistinct cytoplasmic borders (x 400). (B) The same case, showing darkly stained granules filling the cytoplasm of the tumor cells. The nuclei appear as clear discs since no counter stain has been used, (PAS stain, after 80% alcohol fixation, x 400).

In properly fixed material (80% alcohol) stained by the McManus and Hotchkiss techniques, (periodic acid-Schiff [PAS] stain), intracellular glycogen granules, which fill the cytoplasm and vary in size from fine to coarse, may be seen (Figure 12B).[62][63] These are absent in reticulum cell sarcoma and in neuroblastoma, and their presence is therefore an important aid in diagnosis. Most of the tumor cells contain the granules, but in some areas apart from the necrotic zones, glycogen may be lacking. Previous digestion by ptyalin or Taka-diastase causes the PAS-positive granules to disappear, thus confirming that they were indeed glycogen. Periodic acid-Schiff staining without nuclear counterstain is preferable because the glycogen granules are more clearly visible with this technique. Silver stains show a lobular distribution of reticular fibers circumscribing large areas of tumor cells into which few, if any, fibers penetrate (Figure 13).

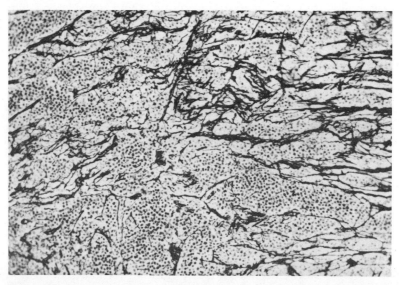

Figure 13 Reticulum stain at low magnification showing the reticulin fibers circumscribing large lobules of tumor cells (Del Rio Hortega's silver technique, x 100).

Formalin preserves glycogen inconstantly, but the latter can still be demonstrated in material fixed in formalin for a long period in about 50% of the cases. Johnson and Pomeroy claim that glycogen was demonstrated in all their cases in which short formalin fixation was used.[64] We have found that the absence of glycogen in material which has been incorrectly treated—either by decalcification in acids or by fixation in formalin for long periods—does not necessarily exclude a diagnosis of Ewing's sarcoma. Several electron microscopic studies have also confirmed the constant finding of cytoplasmic glycogen in Ewing's sarcoma.[65] [66]

There are a few bone tumors that can present diagnostic difficulties due to an abundance of glycogen in their tumor cells. Cells in undifferentiated areas of osteosarcoma may contain glycogen.[16] In these cases, the intense alkaline phosphatase activity of the osteosarcoma tumor cells permits their differentiation from Ewing's sarcoma, in which such activity is absent. Alveolar or embryonal rhabdomyosarcomas, which sometimes invade bone secondarily, may also show abundant cytoplasmic glycogen and other histologic features similar to those of Ewing's sarcoma. Angervall and Enzinger recently have reported a round cell soft tissue tumor with cytologic and histochemical features (ie, abundant cytoplasmic glycogen) such as those of Ewing's sarcoma.[67] In our opinion, however, the tumor described as a distinct entity by Ewing was of medullary origin, and a tumoral process of clearly soft tissue origin should not be accepted as true Ewing's sarcoma—at least not until the histogenesis has been ascertained.

The clinical and, above all, histologic distinction of Ewing's sarcoma from metastatic neuroblastoma, in which the characteristic rosettelike structures are often lacking, may be extremely difficult. Neuroblastoma is more common in children under five years of age. Exophthalmos is often present, and the roentgenographic findings commonly include radiolucent lesions located in the metaphysis of long bones (humerus, femur) or in the skull. In addition, in none of our cases which were correctly fixed was glycogen found. Also, with special silver stains, nerve fibrils can often be demonstrated, and the biochemical study of urinary catecholamine excretion (norepinephrine, epinephrine, and 3-methoxy-4-hydroxymandelic acid, VMA) has been positive in about 80% of the cases.[68] Finally, the most specific and definitive features of neuroblastoma are observed with the electron microscope.[65] This demonstrates the presence of neurosecretory granules and neural processes containing neurofilaments, which also helps to distinguish the tumor from the other round cell sarcomas.

Primary Reticulum Cell Sarcoma and Lymphosarcoma

The term *primary reticulum cell sarcoma* was proposed by Parker and Jackson to distinguish a tumor clinically and pathologically distinct from Ewing's sarcoma which carries a better prognosis.[69] Only cases which at the time of the onset do not show involvement of other areas (with the exception of regional lymph nodes), as revealed by extensive clinical and radiologic studies (including lymphangiography), should be classified as primary reticulum cell sarcoma of bone. Most instances of the Parker and Jackson neoplasm correspond to histiocytic reticulosarcoma and mixed-cell (histiocytic-lymphocytic) malignant lymphoma, as observed in lymph nodes. However, rare cases of undifferentiated reticulum cell sarcoma may also occur. Well-differentiated (lymphocytic) and poorly differentiated (lymphoblastic) lymphomas occurring primarily in bone are extremely rare.

Reticulum cell sarcoma of bone may occur at any age, but it is rare in children and more common in patients over 20. Radiographs generally show an osteolytic lesion without periosteal reactive bone formation.[70]

Histologically the tumor differs from Ewing's sarcoma in that the tumor cells have a more pleomorphic pattern, prominent nucleoli, and better-defined cytoplasmic outlines. In most cases, numerous reticulin fibers surround individual or small groups of cells which lack cytoplasmic glycogen.

GIANT CELL TUMOR

Giant cell tumor, or osteoclastoma, is an aggressive, potentially malignant tumor which occurs most commonly in patients between 20 and 40 years of age. It is very exceptionally seen in patients under 15 years old and is practically nonexistent in children under age 10.[71-73] For this reason, a description of the tumor type will be omitted, but we will describe in detail the group of benign childhood lesions, most of which were previously regarded as giant cell tumors or variants of this disease. Differential diagnosis is important because the benign childhood lesions are associated with a good prognosis after conservative treatment. This contrasts with the more radical therapy (wide excision or segmental resection) which in our opinion is required for a true giant cell tumor.

GIANT CELL LESIONS OF BONE

We have consolidated under this heading a number of benign neoplastic and nonneoplastic lesions which characteristically present with a variable amount of multinucleated giant cells of the osteoclastic type. As mentioned above, most of them have been classified previously as giant cell tumors or variants thereof but are now recognized as distinct entities.[72 74] However, a certain number of cases are still misdiagnosed and classified as genuine giant cell tumors by pathologists with limited bone pathology experience and without knowledge of the patient's clinical and radiologic features (age, location, etc).[73] Derqui has provided an example of the difficulties associated with the diagnosis of giant cell tumor; he cites fifty cases previously classified as giant cell tumors in children which had to be reclassified.[74] Table 3 shows the previous and the present designations for these lesions.

Two other entities which are common in children also show a certain number of giant cells of osteoclast type. They are the solitary

Table 3

Histologic Typing of Primary Bone Tumors and Tumorlike Lesions*

Type	Benign	Malignant	Intermediate or Indeterminate
Bone-forming tumors	Osteoid osteoma Osteoblastoma	Osteosarcoma Juxtacortical osteo- sarcoma	

Cartilage-forming
tumors
	Chondroma
	Osteochondroma
	Chondroblastoma
	Chondromyxoid
	  fibroma
		Chondrosarcoma
		Juxtacortical chondro-
		  sarcoma
		Mesenchymal chondro-
		  sarcoma	

Giant cell tumor	osteoclastoma	osteoclastoma	osteoclastoma

Marrow tumors		Ewing's sarcoma
		Reticulum cell sarcoma
		  of bone
		Lymphosarcoma
		  of bone
		Myeloma	

Vascular tumors	Hemangioma Lymphangioma Glomus tumor	Angiosarcoma	Hemangioendo- thelioma Hemangiopericytoma

Other connective tissue
tumors
	Desmoplastic fibroma
	Lipoma
		Fibrosarcoma
		Liposarcoma
		Malignant
		  mesenchymoma
		Undifferentiated
		  sarcoma	

Other tumors	Chordoma
	"Adamantinoma"
	  of long bones
	Neurilemmoma
	Neurofibroma
		Chordoma
		"Adamantinoma"
		  of long bones
		Neurilemmoma
		Neurofibroma
			Chordoma
			"Adamantinoma"
			  of long bones
			Neurilemmoma
			Neurofibroma

Tumorlike lesions	Solitary bone cyst
	Aneurysmal bone cyst
	Juxta-articular bone
	  cyst
	Metaphyseal fibrous
	  defect
	Eosinophilic
	  granuloma
	Fibrous dysplasia
	Myositis ossificans
	"Brown tumor" of
	  hyperparathyroidism
		Solitary bone cyst
		Aneurysmal bone cyst
		Juxta-articular bone
		  cyst
		Metaphyseal fibrous
		  defect
		Eosinophilic
		  granuloma
		Fibrous dysplasia
		Myositis ossificans
		"Brown tumor" of
		  hyperparathyroidism
			Solitary bone cyst
			Aneurysmal bone cyst
			Juxta-articular bone
			  cyst
			Metaphyseal fibrous
			  defect
			Eosinophilic
			  granuloma
			Fibrous dysplasia
			Myositis ossificans
			"Brown tumor" of
			  hyperparathyroidism

*WHO International Reference Center for the Histological Definition and Classification of Bone Tumors and the Latin-American Registry of Bone Pathology.

(simple or unicameral) bone cyst and eosinophilic granuloma of bone. It is important to establish the correct diagnoses because of their benign characters. As mentioned above, cure may be achieved by conservative treatment, preferably curettage.

Metaphyseal Fibrous Defect

The term *metaphyseal fibrous defect* has been adopted in the WHO classification because it is only descriptive and does not take a position on the continuing discussions on the pathogenesis of the process.[75-77] This explains the different designations applied to the tumor.

The lesion, in our opinion, is definitely nonneoplastic, and we prefer the term *histiocytic xanthogranuloma*. It occurs in the metaphyseal regions of the long bones of growing children and adolescents, most commonly at the lower end of the femur and the upper and lower ends of the tibia. Radiographically, the lesion is located eccentrically and is radiolucent, with well-defined, slightly sclerotic inner borders.[76] [78] Occasionally the process occupies the medullary cavity and the whole diameter of the long bone (fibula, ulna, radius, or even humerus). As growth proceeds, it becomes more separated from the epiphyseal plate and in some cases may disappear spontaneously.

Histologically the lesion is characterized by a fibrous tissue, with a whorled (storiform) pattern, containing hemosiderin pigment and lipid-bearing histiocytes (xanthoma cells) and also a varying number of multinucleated giant cells. Such histologic features are never seen in a fibroma, and for this reason we disagree with the term *nonossifying fibroma* (proposed by Jaffe),[5] formerly called *nonosteogenic fibroma.*[79] At present, the spindle cells in the lesion are interpreted as histiocytes adopting the pose of facultative fibroblasts.[80]

Metaphyseal fibrous defect is usually symptomless and may be discovered after a routine radiographic examination or a pathologic fracture. Only larger lesions may cause pain. Multiple lesions may occur occasionally.

Aneurysmal Bone Cyst

Aneurysmal bone cyst has been described as a distinct clinical and pathologic entity by Jaffe and Lichtenstein.[81-83] It has been regarded previously as a giant cell tumor (atypical or subperiosteal) or, occasionally, as hemangioma and telangiectatic osteogenic sarcoma. The lesion has also been classified as a hemangiomatous bone cyst and as an ossifying subperiosteal hematoma. The term *multilocular hematic bone cyst* may be a more accurate description. The pathogenesis is unknown and it is not clear whether the entity represents a tumoral process or is secondary to some other, preexisting lesion. Thus, cystic changes closely resembling those of aneurysmal bone may be present in cases of chondroblastoma, fibrous dysplasia, giant cell tumor, osteosarcoma, and other lesions.[84-86] However, most aneurysmal bone cysts show no evidence of any such antecedent lesions.

Aneurysmal bone cyst is most common in the teens and twenties.[84] It is usually eccentrically placed, with a "ballooned out" distention of the thinned cortex, but it may be central in location (approximately one-quarter of the cases) (Figure 14). The lesion usually affects the shaft of long bones and the vertebral column and may be confined to a vertebral body. It may also be located mainly in the arch or processes, and not infrequently involves the two adjacent vertebrae. It has also been encountered in various other bones.

The microscopic aspect is rather characteristic, revealing either large or small blood-filled spaces outlined by fibrous septa of different thicknesses which contain newly formed bone or osteoid trabeculae and a variable number of osteoclast giant cells (Figure 15). The differential diagnosis from true giant cell tumors is sometimes difficult, but the gross aspect and the clinical data (age

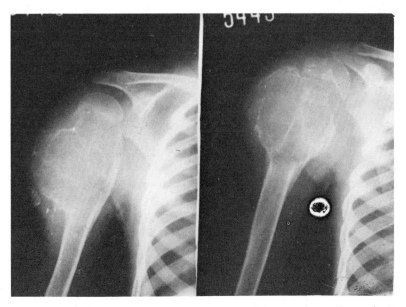

Figure 14 Radiographs of an aneurysmal bone cyst of the upper humeral metaphysis in a 7-year-old boy showing the characteristic "blowout" distention of the cortex.

of patient and location of the lesion) may be very helpful in reaching a final diagnosis.

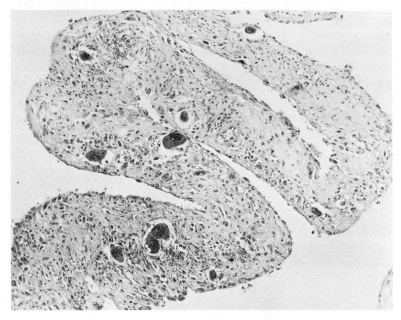

Figure 15 Aneurysmal bone cyst. Photomicrograph showing fibrous septa containing multinucleated giant cells of osteoclast type and some osteoid trabeculae (x 100).

Solitary Bone Cyst

This entity is sometimes confused with giant cell tumor when a certain number of giant cells of the osteoclast type are found by a pathologist who does not have knowledge of its clinical and radiologic features. The histogenesis is uncertain.[87] Solitary bone cysts usually occur in the second decade of life and are located most commonly in the metaphysis of the upper end of the humerus and femur (Figure 16). Histologically it is characterized by a unicameral cavity filled with clear or sanguinous fluid (which is common after a fracture) and surrounded by a membrane of varied thickness. The latter consists of loose vascular connective tissue containing a variable number of osteoclast giant cells, newly formed bone trabeculae, and, often, areas of recent or old hemorrhages or cholesterol clefts. Bands or masses of fibrinoidlike material are frequently present in the tissue of the cyst wall and constitute an important diagnostic feature.[87-91]

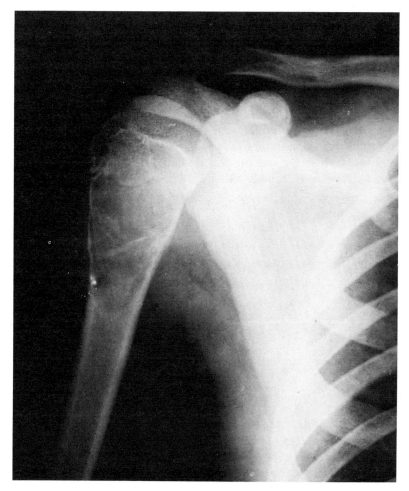

Figure 16 Radiograph showing a solitary bone cyst of the upper metaphysis of the humerus.

EOSINOPHILIC GRANULOMA OF BONE

The concept that eosinophilic granuloma, Hand-Schüller-Christian syndrome, and Letterer-Siwe disease represent different clinical manifestations of a single disorder has gained wide acceptance and has been confirmed by our observations.[92] The terms *eosinophilic granuloma, histiocytosis X, histiocytic granuloma, reticuloendotheliosis,* and others are frequently utilized in discussions of the general disease and its variants.[92-95] However, it has been emphasized that the subdivisions are not sharply defined and that transitional forms between the different entities exist, especially in cases of multiple lesions.

Histologically eosinophilic granuloma is characterized by an intense proliferation of nonneoplastic reticulohistiocytic elements intermingled with a variable amount of eosinophilic leukocytes, neutrophilic leukocytes, lymphocytes, plasma cells, and multinucleated giant cells (Figure 17). Lipid-bearing histiocytes (xanthoma cells) may be found in varying numbers in solitary and multiple lesions but are more abundant in the more extensive or chronic lesions of Hand-Schüller-Christian syndrome.

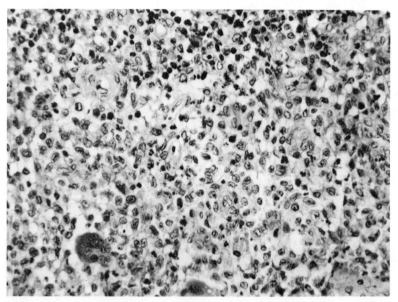

Figure 17 Eosinophilic granuloma of bone. Photomicrograph showing numerous histiocytes with pale ovoid nuclei alternating with (dark) eosinophilic leukocytes and some multinucleated giant cells (x 200).

Children and adolescents are those most often affected, and the most common sites of bone lesions include the skull, femur, ribs, clavicle, mandible, vertebrae, and flat bones. The lesions are osteolytic and may be accompanied by an onion peel–like periosteal reaction in long bones (Figure 18). This makes radiologic distinction from Ewing's sarcoma or osteomyelitis difficult.

Although it is generally impossible to predict the evolution of a particular case from the histologic picture, dissemination of an initially solitary lesion will occur during the early stages—most frequently before the sixth month—and is more common in children under five years of age.[92] According to Enriquez et al and Cheyne, apart from the age of onset, the main difference between the patients who succumb to their disease and those who recover resides in the pattern of involvement of the soft tissues.[96] [97] Widespread dissemination is characterized by a rash and by liver and spleen infiltration. Anemia indicates a grave prognosis.[97] Occasionally, when eosinophil cells are relatively infrequent and histiocytic cells predominate, the histologic differentiation from reticulum cell sarcoma or Hodgkin's disease may present difficulties.

VASCULAR AND OTHER CONNECTIVE TISSUE TUMORS

In general, these are rare neoplasms and are uncommon in children. Many of the benign vascular lesions of bone are multiple and are probably malformations (hamartomas). Other connective tissue tumors, such as desmoplastic fibroma, which is a rare lesion, and fibrosarcoma, which is more common, occur infrequently in children. The few cases of fibrosarcoma we observed in children under 15 years of age were generally very cellular and relatively undifferentiated, with obvious mitotic activity of high-grade malignancy. These lesions usually involve long bones, particularly the lower part of the femur and the upper part of the tibia.

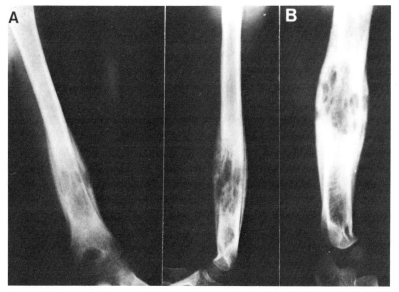

Figure 18 Eosinophilic granuloma: two cases located in the humeral shaft. (A) Radiographs of a 7-year-old boy, anteroposterior and lateral views, showing conspicuous periosteal bone formation simulating osteomyelitis or Ewing's sarcoma. (B) Similar lesion in a boy 2 years old. Both patients are well three years after treatment by curettage.

54

REFERENCES

1. Aegerter, E. and Kirkpatrick, J.: *Orthopedic Diseases: Physiology, Pathology, Radiology.* 4th ed. W.B. Saunders Co., Philadelphia, 1975.

2. Coley, B.L.: *Neoplasms of Bone and Related Conditions: Their Etiology, Pathogenesis, Diagnosis, and Treatment.* Paul B. Hoeber, Inc., New York, 1949.

3. Dahlin, D.C.: *Bone Tumors.* 2nd ed., Charles C Thomas, Springfield, IL, 1967.

4. Fairbanks, T.: *An Atlas of General Affections of the Skeleton.* Churchill Livingstone, Edinburgh, 1951.

5. Jaffe, H.L.: *Tumors and Tumorous Conditions of the Bones and Joints.* Lea & Febiger, Philadelphia, 1958.

6. Johnson, L.C.: A general theory of bone tumors. *Bull NY Acad Med* 29:164–171, 1953.

7. Lichtenstein, L.: *Bone Tumors.* 4th ed. C.V. Mosby, St. Louis, 1971.

8. Netherlands Committee on Bone Tumors: *Radiological Atlas of Bone Tumours.* Vol. 1. The Williams & Wilkins Co., Baltimore, 1966.

9. Spjut, H.L., Dorfman, H.D., Fechner, R.E. et al: *Tumors of Bone and Cartilage.* Armed Forces Institute of Pathology, Atlas of Tumor Pathology, 2nd series, fascicle 5. Washington, DC, 1971.

10. Schajowicz, F., Ackerman, L.V., and Sissons, H.A.: Histological typing of bone tumours. In *International Histological Classification of Tumors, No. 6.* World Health Organization, Geneva, 1972.

11. Ottolenghi, C.E.: Diagnosis of orthopaedic lesions by aspiration biopsy: results of 1,061 punctures. *J Bone Joint Surg* 37A:443–464, 1955.

12. Schajowicz, F. and Derqui, J.C.: Puncture biopsy in lesions of the locomotor system: review of results in 4,050 cases, including 941 vertebral punctures. *Cancer* 21:531–548, 1968.

13. Schajowicz, F. and Hokama, J.: Aspiration (puncture or needle) biopsy in bone lesions. *Recent Results Cancer Res* 54:139–143, 1976.

14. Valls, J., Ottolenghi, C.E., and Schajowicz, F.: Aspiration biopsies in diagnosis of lesions of vertebral bodies. *JAMA* 136:376–382, 1948.

15. Jeffree, G.M. and Price, C.H.G.: Bone tumors and their enzymes. *J Bone Joint Surg* 478:120, 1965.

16. Schajowicz, F. and Cabrini, R.L.: Histochemical studies of bone in normal and pathological conditions (with special reference

to alkaline phosphatase, glycogen and mucopoly saccharides). *J Bone Joint Surg* 368:474, 1954.

17. Jaffe, H.L.: Osteoid osteoma: a benign osteoblastic tumor composed of osteoid and atypical bone. *Arch Surg* 31:709-728, 1935.

18. Jaffe, H.L.: Benign osteoblastoma. *Bull Hosp Joint Dis* 17:141-151, 1956.

19. Lichtenstein, L.: Benign osteoblastoma. *Cancer* 9:1044, 1956.

20. Lichtenstein, L. and Sawyer, W.R.: Benign osteoblastoma: further observations and report of 20 additional cases. *J Bone Joint Surg* 46A:755-765, 1964.

21. Dahlin, D.C. and Johnson, E.W., Jr.: Giant osteoid osteoma. *J Bone Joint Surg* 36A:559-572, 1954.

22. Schajowicz, F. and Lemos, C.: Osteoid osteoma and osteoblastoma: closely related entities of osteoblastic derivation. *Acta Orthop Scand* 41:272-291, 1970.

23. Byers, P.D.: Solitary benign osteoclastic lesions of bone: osteoid osteoma and benign osteoblastoma. *Cancer* 22:43-57, 1968.

24. De Souza Dias, L. and Frost, F.M.: Osteoid osteoma: osteoblastoma. *Cancer* 33:755-765, 1974.

25. Schajowicz, F. and Lemos, C.: Malignant osteoblastoma. *J Bone Joint Surg* 58B:202-211, 1976.

26. Dahlin, D.C. and Coventry, M.B.: Osteogenic sarcoma: a study of 600 cases. *J Bone Joint Surg* 49A:101-110, 1967.

27. McKenna, R.J., Schwinn, C.P., Soong, K.Y. et al: Sarcomata of the osteogenic series (osteosarcoma, fibrosarcoma, chondrosarcoma, parosteal osteogenic sarcoma, and sarcomata arising in abnormal bone): an analysis of 552 cases. *J Bone Joint Surg* 48A:1-26, 1966.

28. Sim, F., Cupps, R., Dahlin, D. et al: Postirradiation sarcoma of bone. *J Bone J Surg* 54A:1479-1489, 1972.

29. Farr, G.H., Huvos, A.G., Marcove, R.C. et al: Telangiectatic osteogenic sarcoma: a review of 28 cases. *Cancer* 34:1150-1158, 1974.

30. Matsuno, T., Unni, K.K., McLoad, R.A. et al: Telangiectatic osteogenic sarcoma. *Cancer* 38:2538-2547, 1976.

31. Fitzgerald, R.D., Dahlin, D.C., and Sim, M.D.: Multiple metachronous osteogenic sarcoma: report of 12 cases with two long-term survivors. *J Bone Joint Surg* 55A:595-605, 1973.

32. Geschickter, C.F. and Copeland, M.M.: Parosteal osteoma of bone: a new entity. *Ann Surg* 133:790-807, 1971.

33. Dwinnell, L.A., Dahlin, D.C., and Ghormley, R.K.: Parosteal (juxtacortical) osteogenic sarcoma. *J Bone Joint Surg* 36A:732-744, 1954.

34. Scaglietti, O. and Calandriello, B.: Ossifying parosteal sarcoma: parosteal osteoma of juxtacortical osteogenic sarcoma. *J Bone Joint Surg* 44A:635–647, 1962.

35. Fairbank, H.A.T.: Dyschondroplasia synonyms: Ollier's disease, multiple enchondroma. *J Bone Joint Surg* 30B:689–708, 1948.

36. Maffucci, A., cited by Bean, W.B.: Dyschondroplasia and hemangiomatosis (Maffucci's syndrome). *Arch Intern Med* 120:544–550, 1958.

37. Ollier, M.: Dyschondroplasia. *Lyon Medicale* 93:23–24, 1900.

38. Jaffe, H.L.: Hereditary multiple exostosis. *Arch Pathol* 36:335–357, 1943.

39. Ehrenfried, A.: Multiple cartilaginous exostoses, hereditary deforming chondrodysplasia. *JAMA* 64:1642–1646, 1915.

40. Schajowicz, F. and Gallardo, H.: Epiphyseal chondroblastoma of bone: a clinicopathological study of 69 cases. *J Bone Joint Surg* 52B:205–226, 1970.

41. Jaffe, H.L. and Lichtenstein, L.: Benign chondroblastoma of bone: a reinterpretation of the so-called calcifying or chondromatous giant cell tumor. *Am J Pathol* 18:969–992, 1942.

42. Codman, E.A.: Epiphyseal chondromatous giant cell tumors of the upper end of the humerus. *Surg Gynecol Obstet* 52:543–548, 1931.

43. Fechner, R.E. and Wilde, H.D.: Chondroblastoma in the metaphysis of the femoral neck: a case report and review of the literature. *J Bone Joint Surg* 56A:413–415, 1974.

44. Dahlin, D.C.: Chondromyxoid fibroma of bone with emphasis on its morphological relationship to benign chondroblastoma. *Cancer* 9:195–203, 1956.

45. Schajowicz, F. and Gallardo, H.: Chondromyxoid fibroma (fibromyxoid chondroma) of bone: clinico-pathological study of 32 cases. *J Bone Joint Surg* 53B:198–216, 1971.

46. Dahlin, D.C. and Ivins, J.C.: Benign chondroblastoma: a study of 125 cases. *Cancer* 30:401–413, 1972.

47. Green, P. and Whittaker, R.P.: Benign chondroblastoma: case report with pulmonary metastasis. *J Bone Joint Surg.* 57A:418–420, 1975.

48. Kahn, L.B., Wood, F.M., and Ackerman, L.V.: Malignant chondroblastoma: report of two cases and review of the literature. *Arch Pathol* 88:371–276, 1969.

49. Sirsat, M.V. and Doctor, V.M.: Benign chondroblastoma of bone: report of a case of malignant transformation. *J Bone Joint Surg* 52B:741–745, 1970.

50. Jaffe, H.L. and Lichtenstein, L.: Chondromyxoid fibroma of bone: a distinctive benign tumor likely to be mistaken especially for chondrosarcoma. *Arch Pathol* 45:541–551, 1948.

51. Bloodgood, J.C.: Bone tumors: myxoma. *Ann Surg* 80:817, 1924.

52. Rahimi, A., Beabout, J.W., Ivins, J.C. et al: Chondromyxoid fibroma: a clinicopathologic study of 76 cases. *Cancer* 30:726–736, 1972.

53. Marcove, R.C., Kambolis, C., Bullough, P.G. et al: Fibromyxoma of bone: a report of 3 cases. *Cancer* 17:1209–1213, 1964.

54. Barnes, R. and Catto, M.: Chondrosarcoma of bone. *J Bone Joint Surg* 48B:729–764, 1966.

55. Dahlin, D.C. and Beabout, J.W.: Dedifferentiation of low-grade chondrosarcomas. *Cancer* 28:461–466, 1971.

56. Schajowicz, F.: Juxtacortical (periosteal chondrosarcoma). *J Bone Joint Surg* 59B:473–480, 1977.

57. Salvador, A.H., Beabout, J.W., and Dahlin, D.C.: Mesenchymal chondrosarcoma: observation of 30 new cases. *Cancer* 28:605–615, 1971.

58. Ewing, J.: Diffuse endothelioma of bone. *Proc NY Pathol Soc* 21:17–24, 1921.

59. Ewing, J.: Further report on endothelial myeloma of bone. *Proc NY Pathol Soc* 24:93–101, 1924.

60. Dahlin, D.C., Coventry, M.D., and Scanlon, P.W.: Ewing's sarcoma: a ciritical analysis of 165 cases. *J Bone Joint Surg* 43A:185–192, 1961.

61. Willis, R.A.: Ewing's sarcoma. In *Pathology of Tumours*. 6th ed. Butterworths & Co., London, 1967, pp 702–703.

62. Schajowicz, F.: Ewing's sarcoma and reticulum cell sarcoma of bone, with special reference to the histochemical demonstration of glycogen as an aid to differential diagnosis. *J Bone Joint Surg* 41A:349–365, 1959.

63. Schajowicz, F.: Differential diagnosis of Ewing's sarcoma in bone. In *Certain Aspects of Neoplasia*. Colston Papers. No. 24. London, Butterworth & Co., 1973, pp 189–202.

64. Johnson, R.E. and Pomeroy, T.C.: Combined modality therapy of Ewing's sarcoma. *Cancer* 35:36–47, 1975.

65. Friedman, B. and Hanaoka, H.: Round cell sarcomas of bone: a light and electron microscopy study. *J Bone Joint Surg* 53A:1118–1136, 1971.

66. Hou-Jensen, P.E. and Dmochowski, M.: Studies on ultrastructure of Ewing's sarcoma of bone. *Cancer* 29:280–286, 1972.

67. Angervall, L. and Enzinger, F.M.: Extraskeletal neoplasm resembling Ewing's sarcoma. *Cancer* 36:240–251, 1975.

68. Voorhess, M. and Gardner, L.I.: Urinary excretion of norepinephrine and 3-methoxy-4-hydroxymandelic acid by children with neuroblastoma. *J Clin Endocrinol Metab* 21:321–335, 1961.

69. Parker, F. and Jackson, H.: Primary reticulum cell sarcoma of bone. *Surg Gynecol Obst* 68:45–53, 1939.

70. Edeiken, J. and Hodes, P.J.: Reticulum cell sarcoma (primary, of bone). In *Roentgen Diagnosis of Diseases,* The Williams & Wilkins Co., Baltimore, 1967, pp 605–615.

71. Dahlin, D.C., Cupps, R.E., and Johnson, E.W., Jr.: Giant cell tumor: a study of 195 cases. *Cancer* 25:1061, 1970.

72. Schajowicz, F.: Giant cell tumors of bone (osteoclastoma): a pathological and histochemical study. *J Bone Joint Surg* 43A:1–29, 1961.

73. Schwinn, C.P.: Differential diagnosis of giant cell lesions of bone. In *Bones and Joints.* International Academy of Pathology Monograph: No. 17. The Williams & Wilkins Co., Baltimore, 1966, pp 236–299.

74. Derqui, J.C.: *Diagnóstico de las osteopatias giganto celulares en la infancia.* Macchi HMS, Buenos Aires, 1962.

75. Campbell, C.J. and Harkess, J.: Fibrous metaphyseal defects of bone. *Surg Gynecol Obstet* 104:329–336, 1957.

76. Cunningham, J.B. and Ackerman, L.V.: Metaphyseal fibrous defects. *J Bone Joint Surg* 38A:797–808, 1956.

77. Hatcher, C.H.: The pathogenesis of localized fibrous lesions in the metaphyses of long bones. *Ann Surg* 122:1016–1030, 1945.

78. Caffey, J.: On fibrous defects in cortical walls of growing tubular bones: their radiologic appearance, structure, prevalence natural course, and diagnostic significance. *Adv Pediatr* 7:13–51, 1955.

79. Jaffe, H.L. and Lichtenstein, L.: Non-osteogenic fibroma of bone. *Am J Pathol* 18:205–221, 1942.

80. Stout, A.P. and Lattes, R.: *Tumors of the Soft Tissues.* Atlas of Tumor Pathology, 2d series, fascicle 5. Armed Forces Institute of Pathology, Washington, DC, 1967.

81. Jaffe, H.L.: Aneurysmal bone cyst. *Bull Hosp Joint Dis* 11:3–13, 1950.

82. Lichtenstein, L.: Aneurysmal bone cyst: a pathological entity commonly mistaken for giant cell tumor and occasionally for hemangioma and osteogenic sarcoma. *Cancer* 3:279–289, 1950.

83. Lichtenstein, L.: Aneurysmal bone cyst: observations on 50 cases. *J Bone Joint Surg* 39A:873–882, 1957.

84. Biesecker, J.L., Marcove, R.C., Huvos, A.G. et al: Aneurysmal bone cyst: a clinicopathological study of 66 cases. *Cancer* 26:615–625, 1970.

85. Buraczewski, J. and Dabska, M.: Pathogenesis of aneurysmal bone cyst: relationship between the aneurysmal bone cyst and fibrous dysplasia of bone. *Cancer* 28:597–604, 1971.

86. Levy, W.M., Miller, A.S., Bonakdarpour, A. et al: Aneurysmal bone cyst secondary to other osseous lesions: report of 57 cases. *Am J Clin Pathol* 63:1–8, 1975.

87. Jaffe, H.L. and Lichtenstein, L.: Solitary unicameral bone cyst. *Arch Surg* 44:1004–1025, 1942.

88. Baker, D.M.: Benign unicameral bone cyst: a study of 45 cases with long-term follow-up. *Clin Orthop* 71:140–151, 1970.

89. Boseker, E.H., Bickel, W.H., and Dahlin, D.C.: A clinicopathologic study of simple unicameral bone cysts. *Surg Gynecol Obstet* 127:550–560, 1968.

90. Neer, C.S., Francis, K.C., Marcove, R.C. et al: Treatment of unicameral bone cyst: a follow-up study of 175 cases. *J Bone Joint Surg* 48A:731–745, 1966.

91. Ottolenghi, C.E., Schajowicz, F., and Raffa, D.: Le kyste osseux essentiel uniloculaire: etude clinique et antomopathologique de 123 cas. *Rev Chir Orthop* 55:287–303, 1964.

92. Schajowicz, F. and Slullitel, J.: Eosinophilic granuloma of bone and its relationship to Hand-Schüller-Christian and Letterer-Siwe syndromes. *J Bone Joint Surg.* 55B:545–565, 1973.

93. Lichtenstein, L.: Histiocytosis 'X' (eosinophilic granuloma of bone, Letterer-Siwe disease and Schüller-Christian disease): further observations of pathological and clinical importance. *J Bone Joint Surg* 46A:76–90, 1964.

94. Jaffe, H.L. and Lichtenstein, L.: Eosinophilic granuloma of bone. *Arch Pathol* 37:99–118, 1944.

95. Lieberman, P.H., Jones, C.R., Dargeon, H.W. et al: A reappraisal of eosinophilic granuloma of bone. Hand-Schüller-Christian syndrome and Letterer-Siwe syndrome. *Medicine* 48:375–400, 1969.

96. Enriquez, P., Dahlin, D.C., Hayles, A.B. et al: Histiocytosis X. *Mayo Clin Proc* 42:88, 1967.

97. Cheyne, C.: Histiocytosis X. *J Bone Joint Surg* 53B:366, 1972.

4 Radiologic Diagnosis of Primary Malignancies of Bone

John A. Kirkpatrick, M.D.
Robert H. Wilkinson, M.D.

The radiologic diagnosis of tumors of bone may be considered from several aspects since bone is a living tissue. This chapter will consider diagnosis by reviewing the basic principles of osseous growth and reaction. Utilizing these data, the radiologic diagnosis will be considered in terms of (1) patterns of destruction and reaction, (2) the nature of the neoplastic matrix, (3) periosteal reaction, and (4) the location of the lesion within a bone. Techniques utilized in the radiologic diagnosis of primary malignancies of bone will also be discussed.

Radiographic examination of the skeleton is in a very real sense the gross pathology of tumors of bone. As an organ and a tissue, bone is uniquely suited to radiographic examination and analysis. Because of its inorganic constituents—calcium and phosphorus—with high atomic numbers, it stands out in sharp relief from both the soft tissues surrounding and within it, which are composed of elements with low atomic numbers. Thus, one has to remember that most of the marrow within the bone, the blood supply to the bone, and the muscle and fat and cartilage adjacent to the bone are of considerably lower radiographic density.

DYNAMIC BALANCE OF BONE

Normal bone represents a balance of osteoclastic and osteoblastic activity—that is, of structural breakdown and replenishment. This turnover occurs at a greater rate in the young, but it continues throughout life. With age, there is a tendency for osteoclysis to predominate, with gradual demineralization of the skeleton, but the form of the bones varies little in health. Because of this natural dynamic balance of bone, it is possible to evaluate the net effect of pathologic processes on the skeleton within a temporal framework and to determine in what manner the normal turnover has been distorted. It is also possible to determine whether the pathology is local or general in extent.

Within limits, the more bone is used or stressed, the more robust it becomes, because increased osteoblastic activity results. Conversely, the less bone is used, the more prominent the osteoclastic effect, and radiographic density of the bone decreases. Of course, these changes take weeks or months to become evident.

Pathologic conditions can be recognized by assessing the alterations of form or density of the bone and estimating the speed with which the change has occurred. While immature bone may bend acutely with sufficient pressure, bone generally does not bend with chronic force. Rather, it remodels, resorbing in response to pressure and forming new bone as the periosteum is displaced and trabeculae are rebuilt along the lines of greatest stress. Thus, one can determine by the orderliness of reformed bone the magnitude and urgency of the deforming pathologic process. In general, the order or disorder discloses the spectrum of the slowness or rapidity of change, or the benignity or malignancy of the lesion.

Slow-growing, or "irritating," processes stimulate new bone formation gently, with slow displacement of the periosteum and realignment of trabeculae. This permits formation of a homogeneous "repair" bone, which blends smoothly into adjacent normal bone. Such leisurely activity, or chronicity, can be confirmed by the pathologist and a diagnosis of benign disease can be expected.

Greater activity near the periosteum, with repeated episodes of displacement of this bone-forming membrane, permits less time for reorganization and results in a more laminated appearance on the radiograph, suggesting a more aggressive process. A still higher degree of lamination is consistent with greater expansion and a more rapid rate of growth. Frank destruction of parts of the repair process indicates even greater rapidity, and the destruction of repair bone at a rate faster than that at which it can be replaced is the hallmark of aggressive, or malignant, disease.

Lesions within bone also allow interpretation of their speed of growth. Here deformity of adjacent bone results from resorption of trabeculae and cortex and, if there is sufficient time, the formation of new margins. Thus, an intact "expanded" margin indicates slower change than an eroded or incomplete margin, which is unable to maintain its bony integrity. Eccentric expansile lesions suggest a less aggressive process (Figure 1); concentric expansion implies a more aggressive process; and the absence of margins indicates even more rapid growth and an increased likelihood of malignant disease. Of course, fractures or biopsy may alter the validity of these criteria.

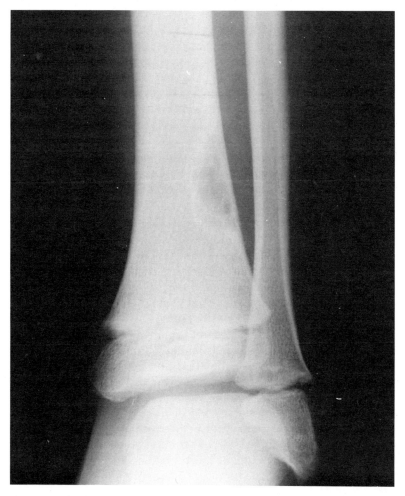

Figure 1. In the distal tibia there is a cortical lucency which does not deform the contour of the bone. The margins are somewhat undulating but are well defined and sclerotic. These features indicate a relatively static process and are radiographic signs of a benign lesion. Diagnosis: benign fibrous cortical defect.

Resorption of bone may result from pressure or hyperemia, or it may follow ischemia. It may be either medullary or cortical. Marrow hyperplasia may cause slow cortical thinning from within, but this would be expected to be generalized throughout the skeleton. Resorption of bone by malignant disease is more commonly focal.

Deformity of adjacent bones is usually associated with an extraosseous lesion, and the rate of deformity and the response of the bones help to estimate the aggressiveness of the underlying disease.

PATTERNS OF BONY DESTRUCTION

The pattern of bony destruction associated with a tumor is dependent upon its biologic behavior—that is, the rapidity with which it grows (its aggressiveness, or "malignancy") and the extent to which the bone in which it arises can contain it. There is undoubtedly a spectrum of such behavior for any one tumor, but certain generalizations can be made. Usually the ability to recognize bone destruction radiographically is dependent upon the physical principles of the examination. A rapidly progressing tumor may produce few alterations in the trabecular pattern of the bone since it spreads through existing channels. With time, of course, the destruction of the cortex as it is penetrated by the tumor will result in a pattern of fine, round or ovoid lucencies which may mimic underlying normal trabeculae (Figure 2).

With penetration of the cortex, a mass of soft tissue may be seen—depending upon its size, the nature of the neoplastic matrix, and the response of the periosteum (Figure 3). If the process is somewhat less rapid, overt bony destruction of trabeculae and cortex will result. The appearance is one of irregular defects of varying size which rapidly become confluent, although islands and/or patches of bone may be bypassed. Again, a mass of soft tissue beyond the confines of the destroyed cortex will be more readily visible if fat planes are distorted, if the matrix is calcified or ossified, and if the periosteal new bone is laminated or destroyed.

When growth is rapid, the transition area between affected bone and normal bone may be most difficult to discern. The slow-growing tumor, however, may result in a large area of destruction surrounded by a well-defined zone of transition. If growth of the tumor is particularly indolent, the edge may be sclerotic and dense, and periosteal new bone will define its outer border if the cortex has been destroyed slowly and time has been allowed for production of new bone. If growth of the tumor is somewhat more rapid, the edge will be well defined, but there may be minimal sclerosis. The presence of septa within the lesion, as is characteristic of chondromyxoid fibroma (Figures 4, 5, 6, and 7), may be dependent upon the rapidity of growth.

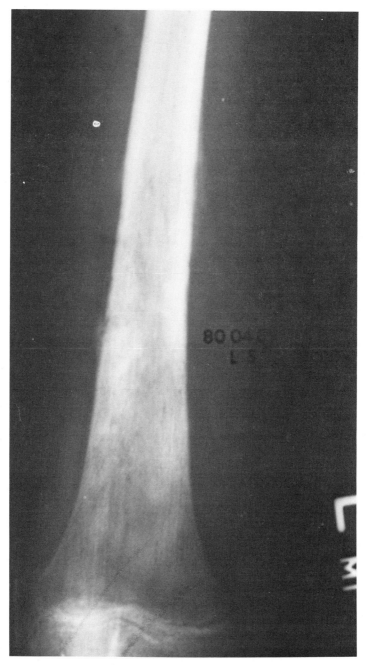

Figure 2. It is difficult, if not impossible, to define the limits of this permeative process. There are ill-defined foci of sclerosis reflecting an ossifying matrix. The periosteal response is laminated and interrupted at the site of a soft tissue mass laterally. These are features of an aggressive neoplasm. Diagnosis: osteosarcoma.

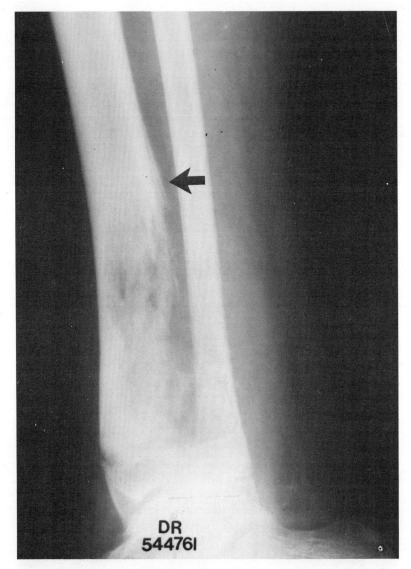

Figure 3. In this tibia a Codman's triangle (arrow) is visible. The pattern of bone destruction is gross but ill-defined. There is a large soft tissue mass posteriorly. Diagnosis: osteosarcoma.

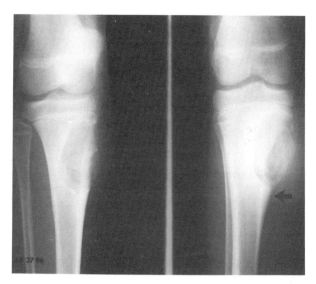

Figure 4. There is an eccentric lytic lesion in the proximal tibia of this young girl. It has destroyed bone locally; periosteal new bone has formed over the outer surface. Note the homogeneous bony buttress at the distal margin where the periosteum rejoins the shaft (arrow). The internal margins are sharply defined and undulating but sclerosis is minimal. This lesion is more active than the lesion illustrated in Figure 1, but it, too, is benign. Diagnosis: chondromyxoid fibroma.

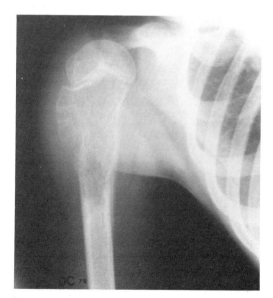

Figure 5. This lesion of the metaphysis extends into the diaphysis, where its margin is distinct but not sclerotic. The lateral margin is covered by a thin shell of periosteal new bone. Medially, the new bone is thicker and intact. There are remnants of normal bone within the matrix. This is a moderately aggressive but benign lesion. Diagnosis: aneurysmal bone cyst.

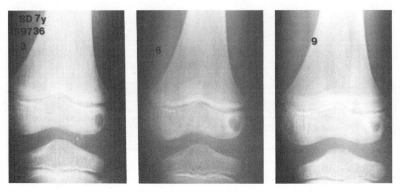

Figure 6. Osteomyelitis in the distal femoral epiphysis shows only destruction of bone in its early, and active, stage. Over the ensuing 6 months, with treatment, bone repair forms a dense margin and the defect is gradually obliterated. Diagnosis: staphylococcal osteomyelitis.

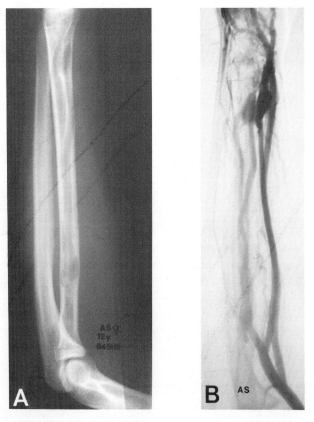

Figure 7. (A) The serpiginous defects in the radius have sharply defined margins, some of which are sclerotic. These represent remodeling of bone in response to chronic pressure associated with this vascular malformation. **(B)** Angiogram showing vascular makeup of the tumor.

MATRIX OF THE TUMOR

As previously noted, the composition of soft tissue is such that it is seen radiographically as relatively uniform areas of intermediate density: any calcification or ossification will be evident. Calcification associated with chondroid tumors tends to be flocculent and in some instances resembles popcorn (Figures 8 and 9). The matrix of osteosarcoma will reflect the dominant type of cell (Figures 10 and 11). If the osteoblast is involved, there may be either isolated, ill-defined clumps of density or an overall, homogeneous increase in density with poorly defined borders (Figure 12). Parosteal sarcoma has a very dense, opaque matrix within its peripheral mass of soft tissue. The margins are well defined and there is little invasion of the bone.

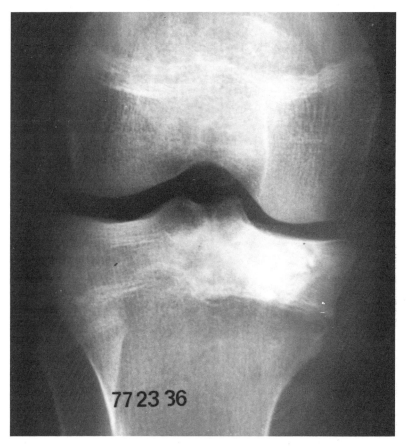

Figure 8. The location of the lesion in the epiphysis of this young man before closure of the epiphyseal plate is significant. Mottled, flocculent calcification is present with the ill-defined area of destruction. Diagnosis: chondroblastoma.

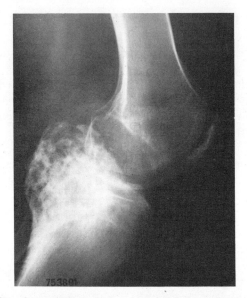

Figure 9. The flocculent calcified matrix is characteristic of chondroid lesions. The tumor is moderately aggressive and has destroyed the cortex posteriorly but is marginated by a shell of periosteal new bone. Incidentally, the process has extended to involve the metaphysis. Diagnosis: chondroblastoma.

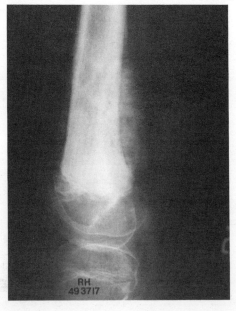

Figure 10. The matrix of this grossly destructive lesion in the distal femur is osseous. Posteriorly, spiculation is relatively coarse, and a limiting shell of periosteal new bone is not present. There is circumferential extension of tumor into the soft tissues. The lesion does not cross the growth plate. Diagnosis: osteosarcoma.

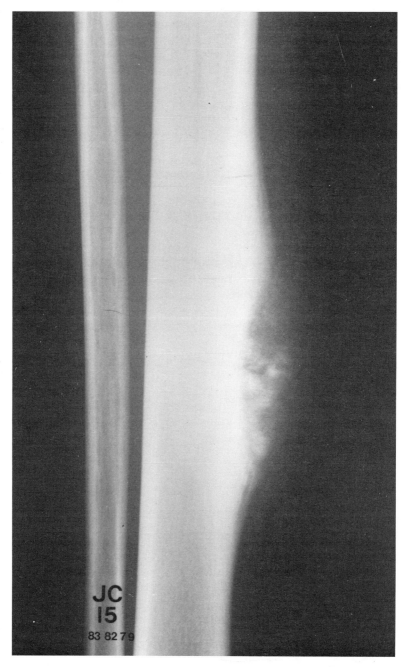

Figure 11. This peripheral, eccentric lesion of the anterior aspect of the distal tibial diaphysis is characterized by a soft tissue mass with a bone-forming matrix. The interrupted periosteal reaction proximally and distally is laminated. Diagnosis: periosteal osteosarcoma.

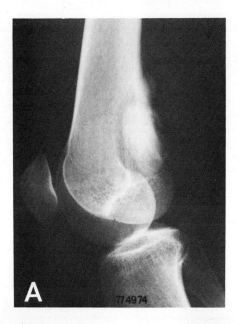

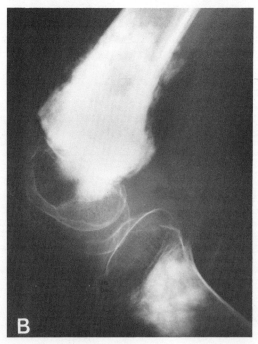

Figure 12. (A) This peripheral and dense, well-marginated and homogeneous osseous matrix of a parosteal osteosarcoma stands in contrast to the osteosarcoma illustrated in B. **(B)** This osteosarcoma is multifocal, sclerotic, invasive, and poorly marginated and extends into the soft tissues at many points.

PERIOSTEAL REACTION

In the event that a tumor destroys the cortex and extends beyond its confines, it inevitably encroaches upon the periosteum to destroy it or cause its elevation. In the latter instance, whether or not it produces visible new bone depends upon the rapidity of the process. In general, slow-growing processess—such as a benign tumor, the edema or pus associated with infection, or blood following a traumatic episode—do not interrupt the periosteal new bone, and a fine, often undulating line or band results (Figures 13 and 14). If the processes are more aggressive, as in Ewing's sarcoma, the initial layer of new bone is penetrated and deposition of a second layer (as the process is repeated) results in a laminated appearance (Figure 15).

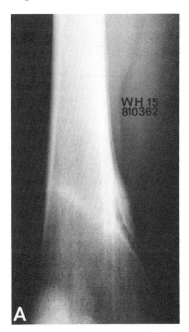 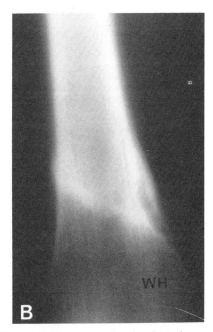

Figure 13. (A) There is mature, dense, circumferential periosteal and endosteal new bone formation in the distal femur of this athletic boy. **(B)** Tomography demonstrates the oblique linear orientation of the well-organized bony repair. Diagnosis: healing stress fracture.

When the periosteum of a limited area is elevated by a tumor, it may be able to respond by depositing a thin shell of bone over the mass of soft tissue (as described above). Localized periosteal elevation, with the periosteum rejoining the cortex and forming a triangle of dense bone, is known as *buttressing* (Figure 4). This triangle of new bone, often laminated, is known as Codman's triangle (Figure 3).

74

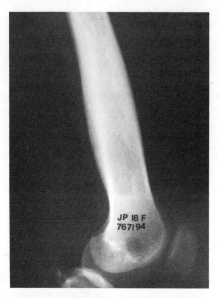

Figure 14. This radiograph shows mature, dense, homogeneous periosteal and endosteal response, primarily indicative of repair, in the femur of an 18-year-old girl. Diagnosis: chronic osteomyelitis.

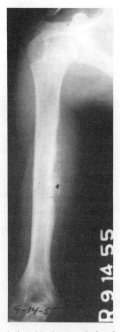

Figure 15. The involvement of the diaphysis of this humerus is characterized by a permeative pattern of destruction. Medially there is penetration of the cortex, with a long area of perpendicular spiculation and patchy destruction of the periosteal response. Diagnosis: Ewing's sarcoma.

However, there may not be time for buttressing, or the periosteum may be destroyed by the rapidly advancing tumor.

A response that may be seen as tumor rapidly penetrates the cortex is the development of spicules, which tend to form at right angles to the cortex. These linear densities may be composed of reactive or neoplastic bone which is presumably deposited about the Sharpey's fibers and the vessels that extend between the periosteum and the cortex. The more rapidly the tumor grows the closer to perpendicular the spicules. Of course, they tend to extend outward from the center of the tumor, and if the locus is limited, as in osteosarcoma, they will look like a sunburst (Figure 10); if the locus is extended, as in Ewing's sarcoma, they will more closely approach being parallel to each other (Figure 15).

LOCATION OF THE TUMOR WITHIN A BONE

It has been shown that many tumors which arise in a long bone involve the metaphyses. There are certain tumors, however, for which location is of significance in differential diagnosis. Ewing's sarcoma, reticulum cell sarcoma, and chondrosarcoma are frequently diaphyseal in location. Unicameral cysts are often encountered in the diaphysis, although many, if not all, arise in the metaphysis and become diaphyseal in location as bone grows away from them. The epiphyseal centers are the expected sites of chondroblastoma, although the epiphyses may also be affected in osteomyelitis and histiocytosis. Osteosarcoma, when multicentric, may also involve the epiphyseal center. It is most uncommon for the primary metaphyseal osteosarcoma to cross the epiphyseal line. After closure of the growth plate, giant cell tumor characteristically involves the end of the bone, the metaphyses, and the epiphyses (Figure 16). A peripheral, cortical site is indicative of paraosteosarcoma, periostealosteosarcoma, juxtacortical chondroma, and, of course, exostosis and peripheral chondrosarcoma. Flat bones may be involved by almost any tumor, benign or malignant.

ROENTGEN TECHNIQUES USED
IN DIAGNOSIS OF BONE TUMORS

A radiographic study of a tumor consists of at least two exposures of the affected part, at right angles to each other. These two projections, of course, may and should be supplemented as needed to define as accurately as possible all of the characteristics of the lesion. Fluoroscopy and oblique projections are readily available. These rather basic studies may be supplemented with more specialized procedures having to do with the particular area of

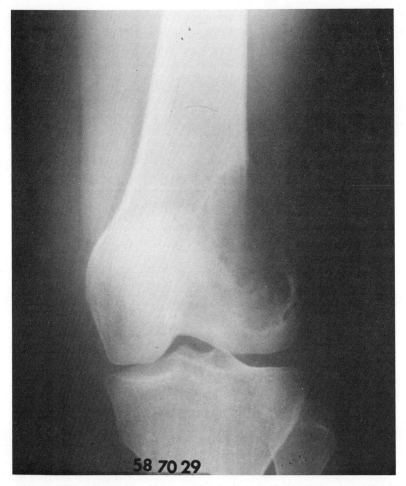

58 70 29

Figure 16. The area of destruction in the distal end of the femur of this young adult is eccentric in location. Its inner aspect is relatively well defined, but its rate of growth is such that the outer shell of periosteal new bone is incomplete and quite thin. Diagnosis: giant cell tumor.

abnormality. It must be noted, however, that examination of the entire skeleton is not to be neglected. Such examination may be a radiologic one, or it may be accomplished by radionuclide scanning, which is more sensitive for the detection of early disease. The finding of other lesions will affect management of the patient and modify the differential diagnosis.

Other roentgen techniques are available. Stereoscopic examination provides a three-dimensional view of a part and allows separation of superimposed structures. It is particularly helpful for the evaluation of lesions of the spine. Laminography is a technique that yields a radiograph of a predetermined layer of tissue

(Figure 13). Multiple such layers may be obtained for examination. Laminography is particularly applicable to analysis of the matrix of osseous lesions and to examination of the detail of the edges of such a lesion. Radiographic magnification is useful for the detailed visualization of the cortex and trabeculae and may be combined with laminography. Arteriography of the skeleton is less applicable to diagnosis than to management of the patient. The extent of the tumor may be determined by its vascularity (Figure 17), and the effects of radiation therapy and chemotherapy may be judged by their effects on the vascularity of a tumor.

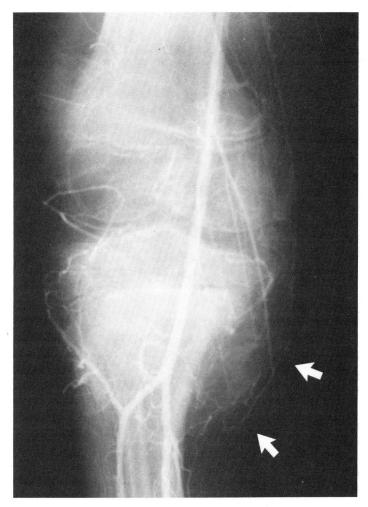

Figure 17. This femoral arteriogram shows the tumor vessels of a neoplasm, which arise in the proximal end of the tibia and delineate the intraosseous and the soft tissue extent of this aggressive process. Diagnosis: osteosarcoma.

In the final analysis, it is integration of the reactions of bone to a neoplasm that permits an appropriate differential diagnosis. Each of the roentgen manifestations has a pathophysiologic basis which when understood will enable their most useful application and interpretation. Their value is, of course, further enhanced by their consideration in relation to other factors, such as age, signs and symptoms, and appropriate laboratory findings. Because radiography reveals gross pathology of bones, it, together with histologic studies, is essential to accurate diagnosis of primary malignancies of bone.

SUGGESTED READING

Aegerter, E. and Kirkpatrick, J.A.: *Orthopedic Diseases: Physiology, Pathology, Radiology.* 4th ed. W.B. Saunders Co., Philadelphia, 1975.

Coley, B.L.: *Neoplasma of Bone.* 2nd ed. Paul B. Hoeber, New York, 1960.

Edeiken, J. and Hodes, P.J.: *Roentgen Diagnosis of Diseases of Bone.* 2nd ed. Vol. 2. The Williams & Wilkins Co., Baltimore, 1973.

Murray, R.O. and Jacobson, H.G.: *The Radiology of Skeletal Disorders.* 2nd ed. The Williams & Wilkins Co., Baltimore, 1971.

Lodwick, G.S.: Solitary malignant tumors of bone: the application of predictor variables in diagnosis. *Sem Roentgenol* 1:293–313, 1966.

Spjut, H.J., Dorfman, H.D., Fechner, R.E. et al: *Tumors of Bone and Cartilage.* Atlas of Tumor Pathology, 2nd series, fascicle 5. Armed Forces Institute of Pathology, Washington, DC, 1970.

5 Scintigraphy in Pediatric Bone Tumors

S. Heyman, M.D.
and S. Treves, M.D.

1. Basic physiology
2. Radiopharmaceuticals
3. Technique
4. Indications for bone scanning
5. Interpretation
   a. Osteosarcoma
   b. Ewing's sarcoma
   c. Malignant lymphomas of bone
   d. Fibrosarcoma
   e. Metastatic tumors
   f. Benign tumors

The value of radioactively labeled bone-seeking agents in demonstrating both structural and functional changes in bone has been appreciated for more than 40 years. The early agents, such as calcium 45 and phosphorus 32, were not clinically useful because external detection of these agents is not possible. With the introduction of strontium 85 in 1942, however, demonstration of both primary and metastatic bone tumors became possible and was accomplished by external counting using a probe. With the advent of the rectilinear scanner in 1951 and the scintillation camera in 1963, imaging could be performed. The quality of bone scanning has improved considerably with technical advances in instrumentation and the development of safer and more suitable radiopharmaceuticals. Pediatric patients may now be studied for both benign and malignant lesions with acceptable doses of absorbed radiation.

This chapter will discuss bone physiology as it relates to scanning, outline the materials and methods currently in use, and discuss the application of bone scanning in the diagnosis and management of primary and metastatic bone disease in children.

BASIC PHYSIOLOGY

Bone consists of an organic matrix which is interpenetrated by a crystalline mineral phase. The matrix is comprised of polymers of glucuronic acid and hexosamines in which collagen filbers, osteocytes, and vascular endothelium are suspended.[1] The inorganic phase is principally a calcium phosphate complex, present in the skeleton as hydroxyapatite $(Ca_{10}(PO_4)_6(OH)_2)$. The crystals are extremely small, measuring approximately 35 nm x 30 nm x 2.5 to 5.0 nm. Therefore, the surface area to volume ratio is large, and this affects the interaction with inorganic ions in the interstitial and vascular compartments.

There are marked differences between the skeletal activity of young, growing animals and that of nongrowing adults. When first formed, bone crystals have a hydration shell, which facilitates the entry of surrounding ions. With maturation, the crystalline structure is perfected, leading to a marked lack of hydration in adult, compact bone. Ion movements are restricted, and a smaller fraction of bone interacts with body fluids. Animal experiments have confirmed a slow equilibration of the crystal interior with the solution phase, which may be distinguished from the rapid, reversible exchange which takes place at the surface.[2]

Bone has a rich blood flow that exceeds the metabolic needs of the tissue. Vessels enter through the nutrient canal and supply the medullary cavity. Radial branches anastomose with the periosteal plexis in the cortex. The outer cortex is supplied with blood from the periosteal vessels, while the inner cortex is supplied by the nutrient artery. Extensive anastomosis exists between the nutrient and metaphyseal arteries.

The incorporation of radiopharmaceuticals into bone is currently throught to depend on both blood flow and possibly two different mechanisms of uptake. These agents may react with inorganic components of bone either by exchange or absorption, or alternatively with various organic components. Examination of tissue slices has shown that radionuclide uptake is dependent on local variations in the state of the bone.[3][4] Blood flow and bone turnover rate are interrelated, so their separate contributions to skeletal uptake cannot be distinguished.[5]

RADIOPHARMACEUTICALS

While methylene diphosphonate labeled with technetium-99m is the bone-scanning agent of choice at present, a variety of radiopharmaceuticals have been used in the past. Of those that have found clinical application, [85]Sr has a long physical half-life (65 days), resulting in high radiation dose. The energy of 510 keV is too high for satisfactory images on the gamma camera. It is no longer used in routine nuclear medical practice.

Strontium 87m can be obtained from an yttrium 87 generator and has a short half-life (2.8 hours). Plasma clearance is relatively slow and the timing of the bone scan after injection of the isotope is complicated by the disparate rates of clearance and radioactive decay. High count rates from nontarget tissues reduce differences between abnormal and normal bone and reduce the diagnostic value of the images obtained.

Fluorine 18 can be produced in a cyclotron or a reactor. It is rapidly excreted by the kidneys and its blood clearance is faster than that of strontium or the technetium complexes. Although the target-to-nontarget activity ratio is high, ^{18}F is a positron-emitter, and the 511-keV gamma rays are not ideal for scintillation camera imaging. In addition, the short half-life (1.85 hours) and absence of a generator system leads to problems in distribution.

Bone scanning in pediatrics has become more widely accepted since the recent advent of the ^{99m}Tc-Sn-phosphorus complexes. These include labeled polyphosphates; pyrophosphates; and diphosphonates such as hydroxyethylidene diphosphonic acid or methylene diphosphonate. The 140-keV gamma emission of ^{99m}Tc is suitable for imaging with both the gamma camera and the rectilinear scanner. Because of its six-hour physical half-life and lack of beta emissions, relatively large amounts may be administered and yield a lower radiation dose than other radionuclides. The whole-body dose ranges from 0.131 rad/mCi in the newborn to 0.011 rad/mCi in the adult, and the dose to the bone ranges from 1.10 rad/mCi to 0.08 rad/mCi. The gonadal dose is higher in the female: 0.561 rad/mCi in the newborn (male: 0.289 rad/mCi), decreasing to 0.046 rad/mCi in the adult (male: 0.034 rad/mCi).[6]

The exact mechanism of uptake of these complexes has not yet been determined. It is possible that the phosphate in the scanning agent chemisorbs on the surface of the apatite crystal, releasing both the tin and the technetium. These would then hydrolyze and deposit either separately or together as hydrated tin oxide and technetium dioxide particles. Another possibility is that an association may occur between reduced ionic species of technetium which have been coordinated to the tin oxide and then absorbed as a unit on the apatite.[7] An advantage of the diphosphonates in this group of complexes is the more rapid blood clearance rate after intravenous injection. This may be explained by the relatively higher level of protein binding which occurs with the polyphosphates and pyrophosphates.

Findings in rachitic rats suggest that ^{99m}Tc-Sn-pyrophosphate may have a greater affinity for immature collagen than for the crystal surface of bone.[8] In the normal bone matrix in vivo it seems unlikely that it is the uncalcified portion of the bone producing localization. However, this may be true of rachitic bone, and further investigations are needed to clarify this possibility.[7]

Although it has not found wide application, gallium citrate Ga 67 has been shown to accumulate in several tumors observed in children, including both primary and metastatic lesions in bone.[9-11] The incorporation into bone is through adsorption by hydroxyapatite, particularly at sites of rapid formation, and, in the case of malignant lesions, perhaps also because of affinity for tumor.[7 10] The whole-body doses range from 1.40 rad/mCi in the newborn to 0.16 rad/mCi in the adult. The dose to the spleen ranges from 8.02 rad/mCi in the newborn to 0.06 rad/mCi in the adult.[6]

In those conditions where the bone marrow is involved, it is possible that marrow scanning with technetium Tc 99m sulfur colloid will demonstrate pathology earlier than will scanning with those agents which concentrate in the cortex.

TECHNIQUE

A dose of 200 µCi/kg Methylene diphosphonate ^{99m}Tc is injected intravenously. No special patient preparation is necessary, though oral fluids are encouraged between the time of injection and the scan. This stimulates voiding and results in a reduced radiation dose to the bladder and gonads. The decreased bladder activity at the time of scanning also ensures less interference when imaging the pelvic bones.

Imaging is commenced two to four hours after injection. The scintillation camera is now generally favored as the imaging device. Whole-body scanning is possible when the instrument is equipped with a special scanning table. With this facility it is common practice to obtain both anterior and posterior projections and special static views of suspicious areas using a high-resolution or pinhole collimator. Because of the need for good spatial resolution in the small patient, we favor multiple high-resolution static images in order to include the whole skeleton and allow further evaluation of suspicious areas with the pinhole collimator. The initial image is obtained of the sternum and anterior thorax and the time needed to accumulate 500k counts is noted. The remaining areas are imaged for equal amounts of time; this facilitates comparison of paired structures of the body.

When bone marrow imaging is performed, technetium Tc 99m

sulfur colloid is injected intravenously in a dose of 100 μCi/kg. After about 30 minutes, 100k images are obtained using the high-resolution collimator.

Gallium scintiscans are performed 24 and 48 hours after intravenous injection of 0.03 mCi of gallium citrate Ga 67; 50k images of the relevant bones are obtained, and paired structures are again compared. When a single-peak technique is used for scanning, the gamma camera should be set for the 92-keV energy peak of ^{67}Ga, and a medium-energy collimator used. However, the images are more satisfactory if the gamma camera has a triple-peak analyzer, so that the three major energy peaks of ^{67}Ga can be utilized.

INDICATIONS FOR BONE SCANNING

While it is probably true that by the time a primary bone tumor produces symptoms the lesion will be evident radiographically, a bone scan should still be performed, as it will not only reveal the extent of the lesion but will also indicate any other sites of involvement. This is of importance in planning therapy and assessing the prognosis.[12] There is much evidence that the bone scan is highly sensitive in this regard: positive scans have belied negative radiographs in up to 30% of cases.[12-14] In children this figure may be as high as 68%.[15] Conversely, negative scans with positive radiographs occur in only a very small number of cases.

Once the diagnosis of a primary or metastatic lesion has been established, we utilize the bone scan to determine the extent of the bone involvement, and we mark the limits over the skin. This may be useful in planning radiotherapy and also in indicating a site for a bone biopsy. It is also used in the preoperative determination of the extent of the tumor and guides the surgeon in regard to the level of transmedullary resection, which is one of the approaches followed in the limb preservation program. There appears to be good correlation between the bone scan, roentgenograms, and histologic evaluation of tumor extent.[16]

Response to therapeutic measures is readily apparent in follow-up studies as reduced uptake in the previously abnormal focus, although, as will be discussed later, reduced or normal uptake does not necessarily indicate healing. Uptake may be inhibited by chemotherapy only to increase once more upon discontinuation of treatment. Local progression or distant metastases will also be detected if present, and bone scanning is useful in long-term follow-up of patients with both osseous and extraosseous malignancies which have a tendency to metastasize to bone. It has been postulated that bone scan may demonstrate pulmonary metastases—even some not seen radiographically—from osteosarcomas.[17] In our experience, however, pulmonary metastases are not commonly detected in bone scans and are earlier and better demonstrated radiographically.

INTERPRETATION

Bone scintigraphy is a sensitive indicator of bone pathology—unlike the x-ray, which requires 30% to 50% decalcification of bone before abnormalities are apparent. While radiographic findings primarily reflect changes in structure, bone scans reflect both structural and functional changes. As discussed earlier, uptake of the radionuclide is influenced by both the vascularity and the rate of formation of bone. It is not surprising then that the appearance of the normal scan varies somewhat with age and stage of development. For example, there is intense uptake in the ends of long bones, and scintigraphic appearance is globular in younger patients and later becomes linear as the epiphyseal plate becomes well defined.

Although it is sensitive, the bone scan, unfortunately, is not specific. Abnormalities may be observed in a wide range of malignant and benign disorders. The malignant lesions include both primary and metastatic tumors. Increased activity occurs in such benign lesions as trauma without fracture, recent fractures, various arthritides, osteomyelitis, cellulitis, increased stress due to abnormal weight-bearing, initially with disuse of a limb, metabolic bone diseases, infarction of bone, and benign tumors.

Less commonly the bone scan will reveal areas of abnormally decreased activity. These may occur with primarily osteolytic lesions with decreased reactive bone tissue and vascularity, in some cases of histiocytosis X, with bone cysts, and with avascular necrosis.[18][19] False-negative bone scans have been observed in adults with disseminated metastatic disease.[20]

The bone scan findings must thus be interpreted in relation to the patient's age and details of the clinical history and physical examination. Correlation with radiographs of any abnormal areas is essential for a more specific diagnosis. It is important to know what therapeutic measures have been taken. Radiation therapy may cause an initial increase in uptake, due to reactive hyperemia, but the late effect is decreased activity within the area of the radiation portal.[21][22] Cytotoxic drugs may also be expected to reduce uptake, not only by the tumor but also by normal bone.

In some cases there may be increased skeletal activity distal to the lesion. This tends to be rather diffuse and is probably due to hyperemia. It should not be confused with extensive tumor involvement.

Bone marrow scans will show areas of decreased uptake when there are lesions present which involve the bone marrow cavity. In such cases, whether the methylene diphosphonate ^{99m}Tc scan is positive or not will depend on whether or not there is cortical involvement.

Osteosarcoma

Osteosarcoma is the most commonly scanned pediatric primary neoplasm of bone. By the time patients become symptomatic there are invariably radiologic changes associated with a strongly positive scan in the primary site. Typically this occurs in the metaphysis of a long bone, particularly about the knee. Scintigraphic images obtained shortly after injection demonstrate marked hyperemia, while the usual two- to four-hour views show the avidity with which the tumor takes up the radiopharmaceutical (Figure 1).[15] Scintigraphy has been found to be more sensitive to bone, but less sensitive than radiographs for the detection of pulmonary lesions.[15][23] Less commonly, in patients with multicentric sclerosing osteosarcoma, there may be multiple areas of abnormal activity. The parosteal or juxtacortical osteosarcoma usually arises beneath the periosteum and does not invade the cortex. In these cases, radiopharmaceutical accumulation appears to be outside the bone.[15]

In planning the management of the disease, it is useful to know the extent of the tumor preoperatively. Our surgeons mark the limits of the abnormal skeletal uptake and use this information to decide on the level of surgical resection. With the patient positioned under the gamma camera and with the aid of the persistence scope, a small radioactive source is used to delineate the tumor boundaries. These are then marked on the skin. Since the radiopharmaceutical uptake extends slightly beyond the tumor limit, marking with the help of bone scintigraphy has an inherent margin of safety.

In one study, both the bone scan and roentgenographic studies correlated well in 12 of 13 cases, and there was no extension of tumor beyond the area of surgical resection. In the single exception, a tumor of the distal femur demonstrated a slight increase in uptake of the radiopharmaceutical throughout the shaft, while the radiographic abnormality was confined to the distal metaphysis. Although pathologic examination had not revealed intramedullary spread, there was marrow necrosis, giant cell infiltration, and granulation tissue.[16]

Bone scans have been useful in the early detection of local recurrence of metastases in patients with osteosarcoma. Bony

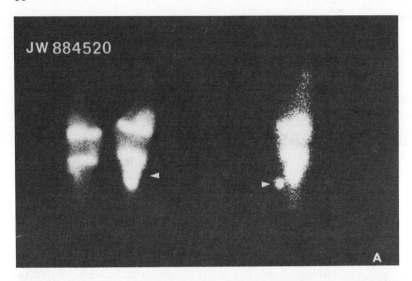

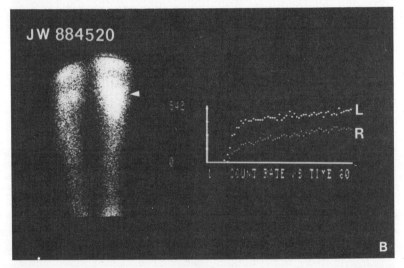

Figure 1 Osteosarcoma, left tibia. (A) The anterior bone scintigram obtained three hours after injection reveals avid uptake of the radiopharmaceutical by the tumor (arrow). On the right of the panel, a radioactive point source is imaged to delimit the most distal portion of the lesion (arrow). (B) Anterior scintigraph obtained immediately after intravenous injection of of methylene diphosphonate ^{99m}Tc demonstrates marked hyperemia in the left proximal tibia (arrow). Time vs activity curves of the upper tibias taken at 0.5-second intervals also reflect the increased vascularity of the lesion in the left tibia.

metastases are not usually seen before the appearance of lung metastases; however, it is possible that, with the increased survival times afforded by newer therapeutic regimens, skeletal metastases may occur before pulmonary involvement in some cases.

In rare instances when radiation therapy is utilized as a primary therapeutic maneuver, there may initially be increased activity within the radiation portal. However, uptake is reduced within three months, and increase uptake in such irradiated areas several months after radiotherapy should suggest tumor recurrence, infection, or pathologic fracture.[23] Where the lower limb has been amputated and a prosthesis fitted, it is usual to find increased activity at the end of the stump and in the region of the ipsilateral hip joint. This is due to increased turnover of bone secondary to the increased stress in these areas. With disuse, the ipsilateral hip will reveal a decrease in radiopharmaceutical uptake. In those cases where the involved bone has been resected and a prosthetic joint inserted, there may be increased uptake in the bone ends for several months after surgery.

While phosphates labeled with ^{99m}Tc are those now used almost exclusively in pediatric bone scanning, there is a possible advantage in scanning with gallium citrate Ga 67 in selected cases. Because of its affinity for tumor and the fact that its uptake is less dependent on bone reaction to the proliferating neoplasm, gallium may delineate the size of the osteosarcoma more accurately.[10]

Ewing's Sarcoma

Ewing's sarcoma avidly accumulates the bone agent (Figure 2). The tumor occurs most frequently in the diaphysis of bones, though less commonly the metaphysis may be involved. As was noted by Ewing, it may also arise in the flat bones of the trunk—such as the pelvis, scapulae, ribs, and skull. Although sarcomas are frequently more hyperemic than benign or traumatic lesions, in general their scintigraphic appearance cannot be distinguished from that of osteomyelitis.[15] Diagnosis depends on correlation with radiographs and other diagnostic procedures. It has been shown that polyphosphate ^{99m}Tc and gallium citrate Ga 67 are as useful as radiography in delineating the primary lesion. Skeletal scanning is, however, significantly superior for detecting bone metastases.[24]

In post-therapy follow-up, the whole-body bone scan should include adequate views of the hands, feet, and skull. The original lesions may either continue to show increased uptake, revert to normal, or actually decrease uptake. The significance of sequential scans showing decreasing uptake is still somewhat doubtful. It is possible that this represents a response to therapy, and that no active tumor remains. However, we have seen such scans become abnormal again while the patient was off therapy, suggesting that the tumor merely had been quiescent and controlled by the chemo-therapeutic agents. While the reappearance of an abnormal focus in

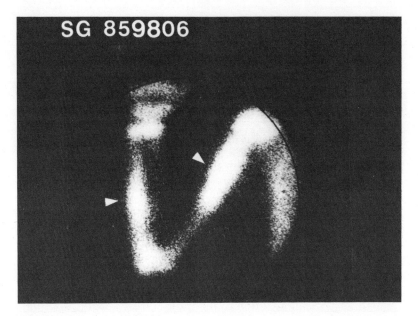

Figure 2 Ewing's sarcoma. There is intense radiopharmaceutical uptake in the right humerus and ulna.

a region which has received curative radiotherapy may indicate either recurrence of disease, fracture, or inflammation, it may also indicate a radiation-induced sarcoma.

Malignant Lymphomas of Bone

A malignant lymphoma of bone may occur at any age, but it is rare in the very young. In a small number of cases there is no evidence of disease elsewhere, and the osseous lesion can be presumed to be primary. Bone scanning has been found to be a more sensitive indicator of disease than roentgenography (Figure 3).[25-27] The neoplastic process is somewhat similar to leukemia in that the bony lesion is secondary to marrow involvement. The skeletal abnormalities may be either multicentric or solitary.[28] It is likely that bone marrow scanning may reveal disease even earlier.

Fibrosarcoma

This malignant tumor does not produce osteoid material, but there may be periosteal new-bone formation. The neoplastic tissue often extends beyond the lytic zone seen in the radiograph. Associated with the reactive bone formation is a marked increase in uptake of the bone agent. As mentioned previously, secondary fibrosarcoma may follow radiotherapy for another lesion. These, too, show increased activity.

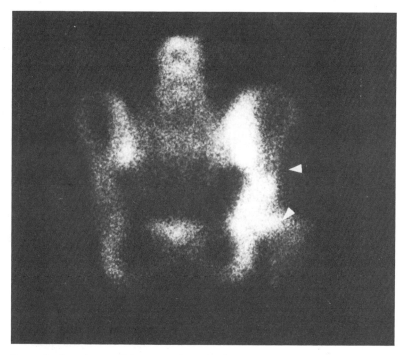

Figure 3 Lymphoma. This posterior image shows increased radiopharmaceutical uptake in the right side of the pelvis due to lymphoma (upper arrow). In addition, there is increased uptake, secondary to a pathologic fracture, in the femoral neck (lower arrow).

Metastatic Tumors

Other primary malignant tumors of bone, such as chondrosarcoma, chordomas, and primitive, multipotential primary sarcoma, are less common. When they do occur, positive scans may be expected if there is associated bony reaction.

Neuroblastoma is the childhood neoplasm which most frequently metastasizes to bone. Metastases are frequently multiple and are seen as increased activity in the metaphyses and adjacent regions.[28] The epiphyses lose their linear appearance and appear as a globular or wedge-shaped increase. Since this may be symmetrical, the scan may appear normal. Thus, great care is necessary in interpreting these studies.[15]

Normal bone scans and roentgenograms do not rule out the presence of tumor cells in the bone marrow.[29] For this reason, bone marrow scanning may be useful for the early detection of metastases (Figure 4). Replacement of normal bone marrow by metastatic neuroblastoma has been demonstrated by reticuloendothelial scanning with technetium Tc 99m sulfur colloid.[30]

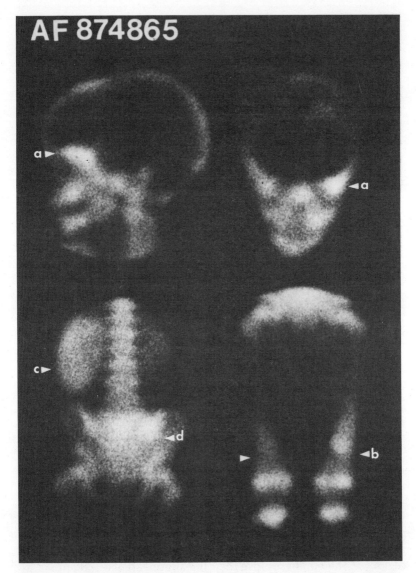

Figure 4 Neuroblastoma with metastatic spread (a) There is increased radiopharmaceutical uptake in the left sphenoidal bone seen on the anterior and left lateral projections. (b) In addition, there is increased activity in both distal femurs, more marked on the left. (c) Also, there is an increase in size and uptake in the left kidney due to obstruction. (d) A biopsy site in the right iliac bone is seen as an area of increased uptake.

Extraosseous uptake of bone-seeking agents by both the primary tumor and by soft-tissue metastases has been shown to occur. These sites may or may not have shown calcification radiologically.[31] Appearance of abnormal activity in the previously normal operation site may be an early indication of recurrent disease. Helson et al's experience with ^{19}F suggests that the detection of metastatic tumors varies with the anatomic site.[29] Lesions in the skull, thorax, knees, or scapulae were more readily detected by scanning than by roentgenography, while roentgenography was better or of equal value for revealing metastases in the vertebral column and long bones. However, experience with the newer radiopharmaceuticals and the modern gamma camera does not support this. Metastases in all sites are more readily detected by scanning than by roentgenography. At present, radiographic skeletal survey, bone and possibly bone marrow scanning, and bone marrow biopsies are all necessary to determine the status of a child with neuroblastoma.

Wilms' tumor   Skeletal metastases with Wilms' tumor are uncommon. However, they can occur, and present as foci of increased activity which are indistinguishable from the many other possible causes of a positive scan. One may speculate that with the increased length of survival now resulting from improved therapeutic regimens, secondary spread to bone may be seen more frequently.

Leukemia   In leukemia, bone scans are obtained to establish whether bone pain is due to an infiltrative process or to osteomyelitis. Both these conditions give rise to increased uptake of radiopharmaceuticals in the involved area. Since the cortical abnormality in leukemia is secondary to marrow involvement, bone marrow scanning may be of greater value than skeletal scintigraphy. An abnormal focus of decreased activity in the marrow scan, when observed in association with a normal bone scan, would suggest leukemic infiltration rather than infection. If, however, the bone scan is also abnormal, no specific conclusion can be drawn.

Rhabdomyosarcoma presents as a mass, most commonly in the head and neck, although it has been reported in almost every area of the body. Both sexes are affected, and the tumor occurs in all age groups. Metastases are frequent and occur not only in lymph nodes, lung, and liver but also in bone and bone marrow. The bone scan shows nonspecific increased activity once spread had occurred (Figure 5).

There are several conditions which, though benign, may simulate primary tumors of bone. While the bone scan appearances are not characteristic, some of the more common lesions are briefly described.

Eosinophilic granuloma   Histiocytosis X includes a spectrum of conditions ranging from the usually solitary eosinophilic granuloma, through the Hand-Schüller-Christian syndrome, to the

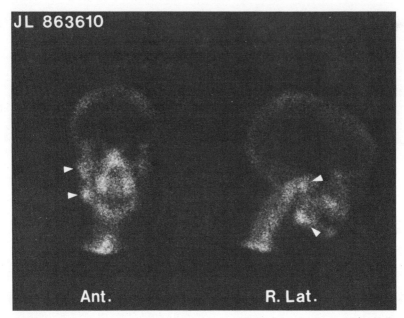

JL 863610

Ant.

R. Lat.

Figure 5 A rhabdomyosarcoma of the right parotid gland showing increased activity in the region of the primary tumor and in the right mandible, seen in the anterior and right lateral projections.

fulminating, rapidly fatal Letterer-Siwe disease. Osseous lesions ordinarily dominate the pathologic picture. It is basically a disease of the reticuloendothelial system. The appearance of the bone scan is variable. When there is expansion of the marrow cavity without cortical involvement, the bone scan may be essentially normal. Marked increase in the uptake of the radiopharmaceutical is seen (1) following pressure necrosis, (2) in the subsequent repair phase of the disease, and (3) in the acute phase, when the lesion is in bone and periosteal stripping has occurred.[32] In one reported series, nine of ten cases of eosinophilic granuloma had abnormal scans, while in our experience, five out of six showed increased activity.[33]

Osteoid osteomas are generally considered to be benign neoplasms. The lesion consists of a nidus often surrounded by a zone of sclerotic bone. The major component is a meshwork of osteoid trabeculae, showing varying degrees of mineralization, in a background of more or less vascular fibrous tissue. Bone pain is the most common complaint, and it is characteristically relieved by salicylates. The bone scan of this condition is usually strongly positive. It has been found to be especially useful in assessing lesions of the hips, spine, or other sites when the radiograph is not definitive. Because of the small size of the tumors, it is often necessary in these cases to obtain pinhole images. The scan is probably least valuable for osteoid osteomas of the long bones, where the radiologic diagnosis is usually definitive.[33]

Fibrous dysplasia is probably the result of an anomaly in the development of bone. There may be one or more discrete skeletal defects. Clinically, the lesions may be asymptomatic but produce defective growth and deformity. The upper femur is most commonly involved. Any other bone may be affected, however, including those of the face and skull. The defects exhibit markedly increased activity in the bone scan, making distinction from malignancy or infection difficult.

Bone cysts The simple, or "unicameral," bone cyst is of unknown cause but apparently results from a disturbance of growth at the epiphyseal line. Most cases occur in the upper diaphysis of the humerus, femur, or tibia. While some patients present with bone pain, most lesions are recognized only after a pathologic fracture. Aneurysmal bone cysts tend to occur in the metaphyseal regions of long bones, but any bone may be affected. These cysts cause pain and swelling. While the surrounding bone in aneurysmal bone cysts accumulates slightly more radiopharmaceutical than normal bone, the simple cysts do not. With suitable collimation, the latter will appear as areas of decreased activity.[32] Those cases which have been subjected to trauma will, however, show increased uptake in the bone.

Giant cell tumors are uncommon in the pediatric age group. The uptake of the radionuclide is usually less than in Ewing's sarcoma and they are generally indistinguishable from other lesions.

Chondrogenic tumors Osteochondroma is the most common of benign bone tumors. A smaller group has numerous lesions affecting many bones. The bone scan is abnormal, showing variable uptake of the radiopharmaceutical, but the radiograph is of greater value in establishing a diagnosis.

Benign chondroblastomas show a moderate degree of increased activity. They generally involve the epiphyses and adjacent metaphyseal regions. Chondromas of bone are benign tumors composed of mature hyaline cartilage. Most commonly they are centrally located in bone and are known as enchondromas.

SUMMARY

The bone scan may be extremely helpful in both the initial evaluation and follow-up of patients with primary and secondary malignancies of bone. At presentation, the localization and delineation of the extent of the tumor is useful for both surgical and radiotherapeutic intervention purposes. Scintigrams during follow-up are useful for assessing response to therapy and for early demonstration of metastatic spread. However, scintigraphic findings are generally nonspecific, and skeletal uptake also occurs in several benign conditions. Interpretation of bone scans must be made in relation to the patient's history, physical findings, radiographs of the involved sites, and the results of other investigative procedures.

REFERENCES

1. Merrick, M.V.: Review article: bone scanning. *Br J Radiol* 48:327–351, 1975.

2. Neuman, W.F. and Neuman, M.W.: The nature of the mineral phase of bone. *Chem Rev* 53:1–45, 1953.

3. Comar, C.L., Lotz, W.E., and Boyd, G.A.: Autoradiographic studies of calcium, strontium, and phosphorus distribution in the bones of the growing pig. *Am J Anat* 90:113–129, 1952.

4. Wood, S.K., Lee, W.R., Shimmins, J. et al: Bone mineralization in the rabbit. In Jeliffe, A.M. and Strickland, B.J. (eds): *Symposium Ossium.* E & S Livingstone, London, 1970, pp 124–126.

5. Brooks, M. and Helal, B.: Vascular factors in osteogenesis. In Jeliffe, A.M. and Strickland, B.J. (eds): *Symposium Ossium.* E & S Livingstone, London, 1970, pp 129–132.

6. Kereiakes, J.G., Feller, P.A., Ascoli, F.A. et al: Pediatric radiopharmaceutical dosimetry. In *Radiopharmaceutical Symposium,* proceedings of conference held at Oak Ridge, Tenn., April 26–29, 1976. US Department of Health, Education, and Welfare, Federal Drug Administration, 1976.

7. Jones, A.G., Francis, M.D., and Davis, M.A.: Bone scanning: radionuclidic reaction mechanisms. *Semin Nucl Med* 6:3–18, 1976.

8. Rosenthall, L. and Kaye, M.: Observations on the mechanism of ^{99m}Tc-labeled phosphate complex uptake in metabolic disease. *Semin Nucl Med* 6:59–67, 1976.

9. Milder, M.S., Glick, J.H., Hendersen, E.S. et al: ^{67}Ga scintigraphy in acute leukemia. *Cancer* 32:803–808, 1973.

10. Okuyama, S., Ito, Y., Awano, T. et al: Prospects of ^{67}Ga scanning in bone neoplasms. *Radiology* 106:123–128, 1973.

11. Handmaker, H. and O'Mara, R.E.: Gallium imaging in pediatrics. *J Nucl Med* 18:1057–1063, 1977.

12. Benoit, F.L.: Whole-body survey scintiscanning for bone metastases, abstructed. *J Nucl Med* 9:303, 1968.

13. O'Mara, R.E.: Bone scanning in osseous metastatic disease. *JAMA* 229:1915–1917, 1974.

14. Desaulniers, M., Lacourciere, Y., Lisbona, R. et al: A detailed comparison of bone scanning with ^{99m}Tc polyphosphate and radiographic skeletal surveys for neoplasm. *J Can Assoc Radiol* 24:340-343, 1973.

15. Gilday, D.L., Ash, J.M., and Reilly, B.J.: Radionuclide skeletal survey for pediatric neoplasms. *Radiology* 123:399-406, 1977.

16. Goldman, A.B., Becker, M.H., Braunstein, P. et al: Bone scanning osteogenic sarcoma: correlation with surgical pathology. *Am J Roentgenol Rad Ther Nucl Med* 124:83-90, 1975.

17. Ghaed, N., Thrall, J.H., Pinsky, S.M. et al: Detection of extraosseous metastases from osteosarcoma with ^{99m}Tc polyphosphate bone scanning. *Radiology* 112:373-375, 1974.

18. Sy, W.M., Westry, D.W., and Weinberger, G.: 'Cold' lesions on bone imaging. *J Nucl Med* 16:1013-1016, 1975.

19. Goergen, T.G., Alazraki, N.P., Halpen, S.E. et al: 'Cold' bone lesions: a newly recognized phenomenon in bone imaging. *J Nucl Med* 15:1120-1124, 1974.

20. Thrupkaew, A.K., Henkin, R.E., and Quinn, J.L.: False-negative bone scans in disseminated metastatic disease. *Radiology* 113:383-386, 1974.

21. Bell, E.G., McAfee, J.G., and Constable, W.C.: Local radiation damage to bone and marrow demonstrated by radioisotope imaging. *Radiology* 92:1083, 1969.

22. Fordham, E.W. and Ramachandran, P.C.: Radionuclide imaging of osseous trauma. *Semin Nucl Med* 15:411, 1974.

23. McNeil, B.J., Cassady, J.R., Geiser, C.F. et al: Fluorine 18 bone scintigraphy in children with osteosarcoma or Ewing's sarcoma. *Radiology* 109:627-631, 1973.

24. Frankel, R.S., Jones, A.E., Cohen, J.A. et al: Clinical correlations of ^{67}Ga and skeletal whole-body radionuclide studies with radiography in Ewing's sarcoma. *Radiology* 110:597-603, 1974.

25. Weber, W.G., Denardo, G.L., and Bergin, J.J.: Scintiscanning in malignant lymphomatous involvement of bone. *Arch Intern Med* 121:433-437, 1968.

26. Harbert, J.C. and Ashburn, W.L.: Radiostrontium bone scanning in Hodgkin's disease. *Cancer* 22:58-63, 1968.

27. Dworkin, H.J. and Filmanowicz, E.V.: Radiofluoride photoscanning of bone in reticulum cell sarcoma. *JAMA* 198:985-988, 1966.

28. Gilday, D.: Nuclear medicine and pediatric neoplasia. *Pediatr Clin North Am* 23:41-53, 1976.

29. Helson, L., Watson, R.C., Benua, R.S. et al: Fluorine 18

radioisotope scanning of metastatic bone lesions in children with neuroblastoma. *Am J Roentgenol* 115:191–199, 1972.

30. Judisch, J.M. and McIntyre, P.A.: Recognition of metastatic neuroblastoma by scanning the reticuloendothelial system (RES). *Johns Hopkins Med J* 130:83–86, 1972.

31. Rosenfield, N. and Treves, S.: Osseous and extraosseous uptake of fluorine 18 and technetium 99m polyphosphate in children with neuroblastoma. *Radiology* 111:127–133, 1974.

32. Bell, E.G., McAfee, J.G., and Mahon, D.F.: Bone scanning. In Schneider, P.B. and Treves, S. (eds): *Nuclear Medicine in Clinical Practice.* Amsterdam: Elsevier, in press.

33. Gilday, D.L. and Ash, J.M.: Benign bone tumors. *Semin Nucl Med* 6:33–46, 1976.

6 Chemotherapy of Ewing's Sarcoma

Wataru W. Sutow, M.D.

In recent years, several integrated programs of adjuvant chemotheraphy and radiation therapy have been tried in Ewing's sarcoma.[1-9] The results of these programs have engendered cautious optimism regarding (a) improvement in the rate of control of the primary lesion, (b) the probability of eradication of distant, occult micrometastases, and (c) palliation of macrometastases. However, unlike the clear-cut demonstration of chemotherapy's significant improvement of the prognosis in children with Wilms' tumor, rhabdomyosarcoma, and osteosarcoma, the impact of present-day chemotherapy on patients with Ewing's sarcoma is still not fully defined.[10,11]

For the most part, the cautious attitude toward this treatment probably arises from the well-known propensity of Ewing's sarcoma for developing late metastases. Pritchard et al report that, in a single institution experience with 229 patients (at the Mayo Clinic), of the 37 patients alive at five years, 6 died of tumor by ten years.[12] Most studies of chemotherapy programs do not provide sufficient follow-up data at five or more years to permit observations of this type.

In this chapter, the specific role of chemotherapy in the broad therapeutic strategy for Ewing's sarcoma will be reviewed. The effectiveness of chemotherapy must be assessed in terms of the objectives to be attained. The objectives in respect to Ewing's sarcoma include the following:

1. Improvement of the rate of local control of the primary tumor;
2. Eradication of subclinical micrometastases, and resultant improvement of the cure rate;
3. Capacity to modify radiation therapy to improve the quality of cure (preservation of normal function);
4. Decrease in the risk of the life-threatening sequelae of therapy (e.g., development of second malignant tumors);
5. Significant palliation or cure of the patient with macrometastases.

COMPARATIVE STUDY OF CURRENT REGIMENS

The adjuvant chemotherapeutic regimens currently used by various investigators for nonmetastatic Ewing's sarcoma are basically structured around combinations of two or more of the following four drugs: vincristine, cyclophosphamide, actinomycin D, and Adriamycin.[13-20] In phase II single-agent drug trials, each of the four drugs has demonstrated antitumor activity in patients with metastatic Ewing's sarcoma. Table 1 summarizes the various combinations used in those studies which provide the most significant data. The regimens listed in Table 1 vary in the doses, scheduling, and sequence of courses, intervals between cycles, and total duration of therapy. For purposes of comparison, the information relative to these individual items is presented in Table 2.

Toxicity

The manifestations of toxicity for each drug used in the various chemotherapy regimens shown in Tables 1 and 2 are well known. However, the severity and the nature of the side effects when the drugs are given in combination, or when they are given in conjunction with radiation, may become critical determinants of the adequacy of the planned therapeutic program. Thus the chemotherapist who participates in the care of a child with Ewing's sarcoma must be

Table 1
Current Chemotherapy Regimens

Hospital	Drug Utilized in Chemotherapy Program				
	Vincristine	Actinomycin D	Cyclophosphamide	Adriamycin	Intrathecal Methotrexate
Memorial Sloan-Kettering[6-9]	+	+	+	+	−
M.D. Anderson[1]	+	−	+	−	−
Sidney Farber[3]	+	+	+	−	−
Intergroup Study[2]	+	+	+	+	−
National Cancer Institute[4,5]	+	+	+	+	+
St. Jude[2]	+	−	+	−	−

Table 2
Drugs, Doses, and Schedules

Regimen	Vincristine	Actinomycin D	Cyclophosphamide	Adriamycin	Comments
Memorial Sloan-Kettering[6-9]	1.5-2.0 mg/M² weekly x 4: on days 42, 49, 56, 63 of each 12-week cycle	450 mcg/M² daily x 5 at start of each 12-week cycle	1200 mg/M² biweekly x 2: on days 42 and 56 of each 12-week cycle	20 mg/M² daily x 3 on days 14 and 28 of each 12-week cycle until cumulative dose, of 500-600 mg/M² is reached	8 cycles over 18-20 months

Table 2 (*continued*)

Regimen	Vincristine	Actinomycin D	Cyclophosphamide	Adriamycin	Comments
M.D. Anderson[1]	2.0 mg/M² weekly x 5 at start of regimen, then 2 doses, a week apart, with each pulse of CYT cyclophosphamide		300 mg/M² daily until wbc drops below 2000/mm³ (maximum of 10 doses). Pulses repeated q 8 weeks x 5		5 cycles over 8-month period
Sidney Farber[3]	2 mg/M² weekly x 12 or more doses if tolerated.	225 mcg/M² daily x 7 q 12 weeks	300 mg/M² daily x 7 q 12 weeks		Treatment administered for 2 years
National Cancer Institute (series 3)[4,5]	0.04-mg/kg single dose on months 1, 2,4, and 6 for 4 courses	10-15 mcg/kg daily x 5. Two courses in months 3 and 5	40-mg/kg single dose on months 1,2,4, and 6 for 4 courses		CNS prophylaxis therapy with whole-brain irradiation (2000 rad/2 weeks) and single-dose (10-15 mg) intrathecal methotrexate
National Cancer Institute (series 4)[4,5]	0.04-mg/kg single dose given with cyclophosphamide on day 21		40-mg/kg single dose given with vincristine on day 21	75-mg/M² single dose on day 1 of each cycle	Same CNS prophylaxis as series 3. 4 cycles q 8 weeks
St. Jude[2]	0.05 mg/kg weekly x 12 with radiotherapy. No further vincristine	75 mcg/kg in 5-8 days q 12 weeks	10 mg/kg daily x 7-10 q 6 weeks		Continued for 2 years

aware of the effect of one treatment modality on another and of one drug on another. The interactions vary with the dose as well as with the schedule and timing of each drug and modality. The major therapy-limiting toxicities of the four drugs most frequently used have been tabulated in Table 3.

Table 3
Major Therapy-Limiting Toxicities of Drugs

Complication	Vincristine	Actino- mycin D	Cyclophos- phamide	Adriamycin
Leukopenia	−	+	+ +	+ + +
Thrombocytopenia	−	+ + +	+	±
Neurotoxicity	+ +	−	−	−
Cardiotoxicity	−	−	+	+ + +
Cystitis	−	−	+ + +	−
Gastrointestinal toxicity	+ +	+ +	+ +	+ +
Cellulitis (local)	+ +	+ +	−	+ +
Erythema	−	+ +	−	−

+ = Mild toxicity; + + = moderate toxicity; + + + = severe toxicity; − = no known toxicity

The impact of radiotherapy on chemotherapy (and vice versa) is particularly significant. When large fields are irradiated, bone marrow depression from combined therapy is prompt, profound, and often prolonged. Pulmonary irradiation which includes the heart is a factor in estimating the risk of cardiotoxicity from Adriamycin. Retreatment of previously irradiated areas must take into consideration the recall erythema (which may be severe) that can be produced by actinomycin D. When the field for radiotherapy impinges on the bladder, the administration of cyclophosphamide must be carefully planned. Vincristine, actinomycin D, and Adriamycin cause severe local reaction, even large areas of ulceration or extravasation. It is obvious that the injection of these drugs should avoid actual or potential radiation fields. The inclusion of large areas of bowel in the portal of radiation may necessitate modification of the scheduling of actinomycin D and, possibly, that of vincristine.

Results

A compilation (Table 4) of the results reported from several series reveals two major deficiencies: the number of patients treated uniformly in any series is small, and the durations of follow-up are inadequate. None of the chemotherapy series shows an actual median follow-up of five years. Nevertheless, the trend seems to indicate that the use of chemotherapy has improved survival statistics.

Table 4
Results of Adjuvant Chemotherapy Programs

Institution	Patients Metastasis-Free at Start of Treatment	Patients Currently Disease-Free	Duration of Follow-up
Memorial Sloan-Kettering[6-9]	20	15	24+ to 75+ months (median: 40+ months); actuarial disease-free survival: 76%
M.D. Anderson[1]	19	6	12+ to 46+ months (median: 34+ months
Sidney Farber (update)[3]	10	7	6+ to 60+ months (median: 40+ months)
National Cancer Institute[4,5]	43		Actuarial disease-free survival: 64% at 2 years 52% at 3 years
St. Jude[2]	15	10	4+ to 91+ months (median: 20+ months)

CONTROL OF PRIMARY TUMOR

Not all reported series provide sufficient data to assess the effect of chemotherapy on the rate of control of the primary tumor. Such an evaluation is further complicated by variations in the radiation doses and chemotherapy regimens used by various investigators. Chabora et al and Tefft et al have summarized the experience at Memorial Sloan-Kettering Cancer Center,[21,22] where intensive adjuvant chemotherapy (T-2 program) has been administered since 1970.[6-9] Of 20 patients treated in the T-2 program, 18 (90%) achieved local control. The follow-up periods ranged from 12 to 64 months, with a median of 36 months. There was a tendency which implied that, as more time passed, other patients might relapse locally. Figuring statistics on a subgroup of these 20 patients, the same authors found that 11 of 17 patients (65%) maintained local control of tumor for from 11 to 65 months (median: 27 months).

Fernandez et al reviewed the data from M.D. Anderson Hospital, where the local control rates were 52% (19 of 40 patients) in those treated with radiation therapy alone and 95% (19 of 20) in patients treated with an integrated program of high-dose radiation therapy and chemotherapy.[1] Thus, in spite of the relatively small numbers, available data suggest that sustained programs of combined radiation therapy and chemotherapy have virtually eliminated the control of the primary lesion as a therapeutic problem.

CHEMOTHERAPEUTIC MANAGEMENT OF METASTATIC CASES

The selection of chemotherapy for, and its effectiveness in, the management of patients with metastatic disease depend on the nature and extent of any chemotherapy that may have been administered prior to the development of the metastases. When metastases are present at diagnosis, the treatment plan incorporates the same regimen used in nonmetastatic situations. If some or all of the effective drugs have been administered already, the subsequent treatment plan must be individualized.

Three-week cycles of Adriamycin (45 to 60 mg/M^2 on day 1) in combination with dacarbazine (DTIC) (200 to 250 mg/M^2 daily on days 1 through 5) have shown promising results.[17,18,23] Other drugs that have produced variably successful responses are: carmustine (BCNU), daunorubicin, and mithramycin.[24-26]

Even in patients who have not had prior chemotherapy and who are found to have metastases at diagnosis, the outlook for survival is grim. Rosen reports that seven of eight such patients have died when treated on the T-2 protocol, even though they achieved complete remissions for a time.[8] Johnson and Pomeroy report a somewhat more optimistic figure of 31% survival at three years for patients treated under integrated programs of chemotherapy and radiation therapy.[4] Utilizing vincristine, cyclophosphamide, and actinomycin D (see Table 2), Jaffe has treated five patients presenting with metastases at diagnosis, and all five have died.[3]

FUTURE GOALS

Although chemotherapy has contributed some therapeutic advantages, satisfactory control of Ewing's sarcoma has not yet been attained. Treatment failures occur (1) if the tumor relapses locally; (2) if distant metastases develop; (3) if the side effects of therapy preclude normal function; or (4) if treatment itself creates life-threatening problems (such as cardiomyopathy or a second malignant neoplasm).

There are a number of goals toward which advances in

chemotherapy must be directed.

1. Although the control rate of the local primary tumor can be impressively high (90% to 95%), the cure rate still needs improvement. The intensification of drug treatment by manipulating dose, schedule, timing, and combinations may be reaching its limits, and the development of additional effective chemotherapeutic agents is needed.

2. New strategies for the integrated use of drugs and irradiation also require exploration. Effective chemotherapy might permit modifications in radiation doses and/or treatment fields.

3. If maximum control of the primary tumor is being approached, then efforts should be directed toward reducing the frequency of occurrence of treatment sequelae such as functional failures and secondary malignancies. It has been estimated that 12% of survivors of childhood cancer will develop new malignancies within 20 years of their first cure.[27]

4. Satisfactory treatment of metastases still remains a significant therapeutic obstacle, and continued efforts to improve the outlook for these patients are obligatory.

REFERENCES

1. Fernandez, C.H., Lindberg, R.D., Sutow, W.W. et al: Localized Ewing's sarcoma: treatment and results. *Cancer* 34:143–148, 1974.

2. Hustu, H.O., Pinkel, D., and Pratt, C.B.: Treatment of clinically localized Ewing's sarcoma with radiotherapy and combination chemotherapy. *Cancer* 30:1522–1527, 1972.

3. Jaffe, N., Traggis, D., Salian, S. et al: Improved outlook for Ewing's sarcoma with combination chemotherapy (vincristine, actinomycin D, and cyclophosphamide) and radiation therapy. *Cancer* 38:1925–1930, 1976.

4. Johnson, R.E. and Pomeroy, T.C.: Evaluation of therapeutic results in Ewing's sarcoma. *Am J Roentgenol* 123:583–587, 1975.

5. Pomeroy, T.C. and Johnson, R.E.: Combined modality therapy of Ewing's sarcoma. *Cancer* 35:36–47, 1975.

6. Rosen, G.: Management of malignant bone tumors in children and adolescents. *Pediatr Clinc North Am* 23:183–213, 1976.

7. Rosen, G.: Multidisciplinary management of Ewing's sarcoma. In Donaldson, M.H. and Seydel, H.G. (eds): *Trends in Childhood Cancer*. John Wiley & Sons, Inc., New York, 1976, pp 89–106.

8. Rosen, G.: Past experiences and future considerations with T-2 chemotherapy in the treatment of Ewing's sarcoma. In M.D. Anderson Hospital: *Current Concepts in the Management of Primary Bone and Soft Tissue Tumors.* Year Book Medical Publishers, Inc., Chicago, forthcoming.

9. Rosen, G., Wollner, N., Tan, C. et al: Disease-free survival in children with Ewing's sarcoma treated with radiation therapy and adjuvant four-drug sequential chemotherapy. *Cancer* 33:384–393, 1974.

10. Sutow, W.W.: Chemotherapy in the management of childhood solid tumors. In M.D. Anderson Hospital: *Cancer Chemotherapy: Fundamental Concepts and Recent Advances.* Year Book Medical Publishers, Inc., Chicago, 1975, pp 203–214

11. Burchenal, J.H.: Adjuvant therapy: theory, practice, and potential. *Cancer* 37:46–57, 1976.

12. Pritchard, D.J., Dahlin, D.C., Dauphine, R.T. et al: Ewing's sarcoma: a clinicopathologic and statistical analysis of patients surviving five years or longer. *J Bone Joint Surg* 57-A:10–16, 1975.

13. Sutow, W.W.: Vincristine (NSC-67574) therapy for malignant solid tumors in children (except Wilms' tumor). *Cancer Chemother Rep* 52:485–487, 1968.

14. Sutow, W.W. and Sullivan, M.P.: Cyclophosphamide therapy in children with Ewing's sarcoma. *Cancer Chemother Rep* 23:55–60, 1962.

15. Senyszyn, J.J., Johnson, R.E., and Curran, R.E.: Treatment of metastatic Ewing's sarcoma with actinomycin D (NSC-3053). *Cancer Chemother Rep* 54:103–107, 1970.

16. Tan, C.T., Dargeon, H.W., and Burchenal, J.H.: Effect of actinomycin D on cancer in childhood. *Pediatrics* 24:544–561, 1959.

17. Gottlieb, J.A., Baker, L.H., Quagliana, J.M. et al: Chemotherapy of sarcomas with a combination of Adriamycin and dimethyl triazeno imidazole carboxamide. *Cancer* 30:1632–1638, 1972.

18. Gottlieb, J.A., Baker, L.H., Burgess, M.A., et al: Sarcoma chemotherapy. In M.D. Anderson Hospital: *Cancer Chemotherapy: Fundamental Concepts and Recent Advances.* Year Book Medical Publishers Inc., Chicago, 1975, pp 445–454.

19. Oldham, R.K. and Pomeroy, T.C.: Treatment of Ewing's sarcoma with Adriamycin (NSC-123127). *Cancer Chemother Rep* 56:635–639, 1972.

20. Tan, C., Etcubanas, E., Wollner, N. et al: Adriamycin: an antitumor antibiotic in the treatment of neoplastic diseases. *Cancer* 32:9–17, 1973.

21. Chabora, B., Rosen, G., Cham, W. et al: Radiotherapy of Ewing's sarcoma: local control with and without intensive chemotherapy. *Radiology* 120:667–671, 1976.

22. Tefft, M., Chabora, B., and Rosen, G.: Radiation in bone sarcoma, re-evaluation in the era of intensive systemic chemotherapy. *Cancer* 39:806–816, 1977.

23. Cangir, A., Morgan, S.K., Land, V.J. et al: Combination chemotherapy with Adriamycin (NSC-123127) and dimethyl triazeno imidazole carboxamide (DTIC) (NSC-45388) in children with metastatic solid tumors. *Med Pediatr Oncol* 2:183–190, 1976.

24. Palma, J., Gailani, S., Freeman, A. et al: Treatment of metastatic Ewing's sarcoma with BCNU. *Cancer* 30:909–913, 1972.

25. Sutow, W.W., Vietti, T.J., Fernbach, D.J. et al: Evaluation of chemotherapy in children with metastatic Ewing's sarcoma and osteogenic sarcoma. *Cancer Chemother Rep* 55:67–78, 1971.

26. Kofman, S., Perlia, C.P., and Economou, S.G.: Mithramycin in the treatment of metastatic Ewing's sarcoma. *Cancer* 31:889–893, 1973.

27. Li, F.P.: Follow-up of survivors of childhood cancer. *Cancer* 39:1776–1778, 1977.

7 Chemotherapy of Malignant Spindle Cell Sarcomas of Bone

Gerald Rosen, M.D.
and Norman Jaffe, M.B. Bch., Dip. Paed.

The category of malignant spindle cell sarcomas of bone includes osteosarcoma, chondrosarcoma, fibrosarcoma, malignant fibrous histiocytoma, and malignant giant cell tumors. These tumors are relatively refractory to radiation therapy and conventional chemotherapeutic agents. They may appear in a relatively non-malignant form such as parosteal osteosarcoma or as the majority of giant cell tumors found in late adolescence. However, the diagnosis of a low-grade malignant spindle cell sarcoma such as parosteal osteosarcoma depends upon careful histologic examination of biopsy sections by a pathologist experienced in grading such tumors. The treatment and ultimate prognosis depends upon the tumor's grade of malignancy.[1] Roentgenographic appearance alone is not sufficient for diagnosis of a spindle cell sarcoma of low-grade malignancy. The primary tumor is usually treated by surgical abla-tion. However, with the exception of the rare parosteal osteosar-coma, the occasional low-grade malignant fibrous histiocytomas, and the majority of giant cell tumors found in late adolescence, most spindle cell sarcomas of bone are frankly malignant, and both surgical ablation and systemic chemotherapy are essential in their management.

RATIONALE FOR THE ADMINISTRATION OF CHEMOTHERAPY

Spindle cell sarcomas most commonly metastasize to the lungs and other bones. The majority of untreated patients with osteosarcoma, for example, will develop grossly evident metastases in the lungs within one year of diagnosis and surgical removal of the primary tumor. Therefore, all of these patients should be treated with systemic chemotherapy.

Approximately 2% to 5% of patients with osteosarcoma present with multiple bony involvement. This multifocal variant usually occurs in younger age groups and has a very rapid proliferative course (Figure 1). Patients in these categories should be treated on an individual basis. Generally, however, metastases which appear early (within nine months of diagnosis) are optimally treated with intensive chemotherapy; lesions which fail to respond are removed surgically. Metastases which appear after nine months have usually failed to respond to intensive chemotherapy; they are usually more amenable to surgical resection. After surgery, chemotherapy should be considered on an "adjuvant" basis for 18–26 months.

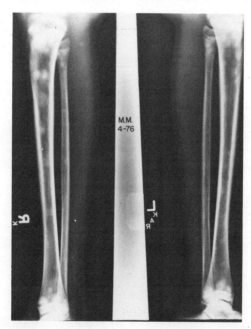

Figure 1   Roentenogram of the leg of a 9-year-old female presenting with multicentric sclerosing osteosarcoma. Note the blastic lesions in the proximal and distal tibial metaphyses and in the proximal metaphysis of the fibula. Leions were noted in all of the long bones of this patient, as well as in the metacarpals of the hand and metatarsals of the foot. She initially presented with a 2 x 2 cm lump in the breast which was biopsied and reported to be sclerosing osteosarcoma.

Systemic chemotherapy probably exerts its maximum effect against microscopic tumor. Even when the tumor burden is small, agents should be administered in doses which are maximally effective against grossly demonstrable disease. Multiple agents are preferable to single-agent therapy.[2] The early application of systemic chemotherapy when the tumor burden is small also derives its support from clinical and experimental investigations. Thus, the survival of animals bearing transplanted tumors is related to the quantity of tumor cells inoculated or surviving after treatment; the larger the number of cells inoculated, the shorter the survival.[3][4] Effective chemotherapy administered under these conditions has produced impressive increases in survival and higher percentages of cures.[5-9]

A metastatis which is sufficiently large to be seen on roentgenographic examination of the chest has a radius of approximately 1.0 cm. At this stage there are about one billion cancer cells in the metastatic tumor nodule. A tumor nodule that is 1.0 cu cm in volume contains approximately 10^{12} cu microns. Assuming the diameter of the malignant cancer cell to be about 5 to 10 microns, some one billion cancer cells will reside in a tumor nodule with a volume of a 1.0 cu cm.[10] If systemic chemotherapy destroys 99.9% of tumor cells, it would still leave approximately one million cancer cells in what was once a visible nodule, although the latter may no longer be visible on roentgenographic examination. Following cessation of chemotherapy, this residual nidus could potentially regrow. Consequently, the eventual surgical debridement of once grossly detectable disease is advisable, if at all possible, prior to continued treatment with systemic chemotherapy. The duration of treatment is still undetermined but most investigators generally consider a one to two year period sufficient for eradication of residual microscopic disease.

CHEMOTHERAPY OF OSTEOSARCOMA

The first major advance in the treatment of this disease occurred with the demonstration that massive doses of methotrexate (MTX) followed by folinic acid ["citrovsorum factor rescue" (CF)] were effective in patients treated for metastatic disease.[11][12] CF is the end product of the enzymatic reaction inhibited by MTX (Figure 2). This form of therapy is difficult to provide effectively and safely, since patients are treated with lethal doses of MTX of the order of 7.5 gm/m² to 12 gm/m², or even greater. Pretreatment with vincristine is administered to decrease the efflux of MTX from tumor cells.[13]

It has been well demonstrated in treating patients with metastatic disease and primary tumors that the effective dose of

SCHEMATIC REPRESENTATION OF FOLATE METABOLISM

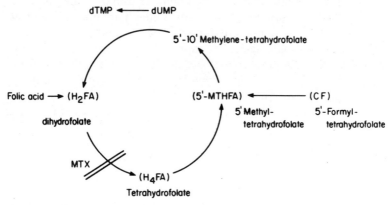

Figure 2 Schematic representation of the mechanism of action of MTX which inhibits the enzyme dihydrofolate reductase, and the reversal of the effect of MTX by citrovorum factor which is the end product of the enzymatic reduction inhibited by MTX.

MTX needed to achieve gross tumor regression is 7.5 gm/m² or more.[11][12][14-17] Further, in the experience of one of the authors (G.R.), the effective dose in young children, ie, those under 12 years of age, is closer to 12 gm/m². The dose of 7.5-8 gm/m² was shown to be effective primarily in the treatment of larger adolescent patients. Extrapolation of this dose to a child under 12 years of age usually results in inadequate therapy when one is observing the effects of MTX on evaluable metastatic tumor. It should be noted that these large doses are needed to cause tumor destruction, and it is senseless to use one-half or one-quarter of such doses in the hope of averting toxicity. Such smaller doses will result in ineffective antitumor activity without reduction in the potentially lethal toxicity.

During the past five years, a number of MTX-CF regimens have been devised at the Sidney Farber Cancer Institute (SFCI), the Children's Hospital Medical Center (CHMC), and Memorial Sloan-Kettering Cancer Center (MSKCC) for the treatment of osteosarcoma. The regimens are illustrated in Figures 3 and 4, and the results in Figures 5 and 6. The long-term overall actuarial disease-free survival varies from 42% to 60%. This compares very favorably with historical control subjects where optimum survival rarely exceeded 20% without the use of systemic chemotherapy.

MTX is more soluble in an alkaline medium. This has prompted most investigators to administer intravenous or oral sodium bicarbonate to alkalinize the urine with MTX-CF treatments.[18-20] Alkalinization, however, was not employed in the original investigations and is not utilized to treat patients with osteosarcoma at the SFCI and CHMC.[11] [12] Patients require very careful monitoring of fluid intake and output to ensure adequate hydration for MTX excretion.[18] [19] [21] A minimum fluid intake of 3L/m²/24 hours is recommended.[21] If the urine is alkalinized, an output of 2000 ml/m²/24 hours for at least 72 hours following MTX infusion is required to prevent toxicity.

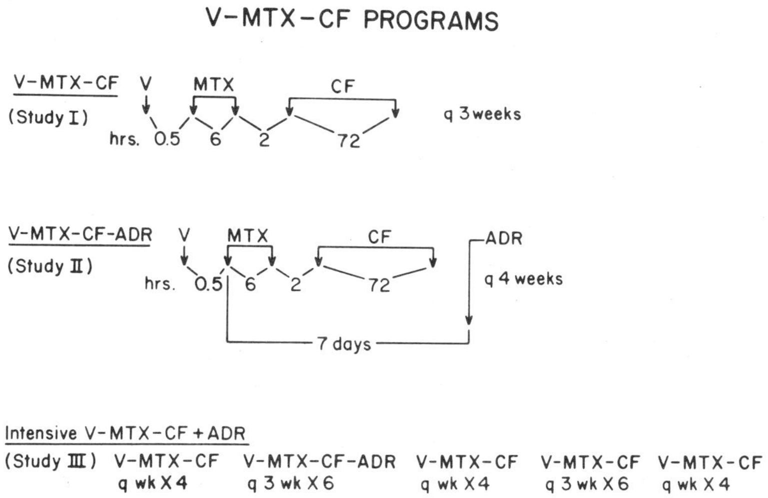

V–MTX–CF PROGRAMS

Figure 3 High-dose methotrexate regimens investigated at the Sidney Farber Cancer Institute:

V = vincristine: 2 mg/m² (maximum 2 mg).

MTX = methotrexate. In Studies 1 and 2, the doses were 3, 6, and 7.5 gm/m² (1st, 2nd, and subsequent doses, respectively).

CF = citrovorum factor: 15 mg q3h I.V. for 24 hours and q6h for the subsequent 48 hours. The first oral dose commences 3 hours after the last I.V. dose.

ADR = adriamycin: 75 mg/m² (maximum cumulative dose = 450 mg/m²).

In Study 2, ADR was administered 7 days after initiation of the MTX infusion. Study 3 represents the current protocol. It incorporates the principles of "front-loading" and reinforcement therapy as administered by weekly V-MTX-CF. ADR is administered 6 days after MTX and at intervals of 3 rather than 4 weeks as in Study 2. The maximum cumulative dose of ADR is 450 mg/m². In Studies 1 and 2, the duration of treatment varied from 18 to 24 months. In Study 3, because of more aggressive treatment, the duration of treatment has been limited to 12 months.

Other chemotherapeutic agents which have been shown to be effective in the treatment of osteosarcoma include adriamycin, alkylating agents such as L-phenylalanine mustard (L-PAM), mitomycin C, cyclophosphamide, cis-dichlorodiammine platinum (II), and combinations of alkylating agents including cyclophosphamide and cis-dichlorodiammine platinum (II) and nitrosoureas.[22-30] Representative examples of chemotherapeutic programs utilized in many of the major cancer centers throughout the United States are outlined in Table 1.[17] [20] [30-32] [34-50] Most investigators experienced in the treatment of osteosarcoma, however, find MTX-CF to be the most effective treatment.[11] [12] [17] [30] [31] Its administration alone or in combination with other agents has produced tumor destruction and in an adjuval setting has improved disease-free survival as compared to historical controls.[32] [33] [51]

The safe administration of MTX-CF is dependent on the integrity of the patient's renal function. Therefore, it is extremely dangerous to combine MTX-CF with agents which are potentially toxic to the kidney. The recent report of the use of cis-dichlorodiammine platinum (II) in patients with metastatic osteosarcoma has prompted

T-7 Chemotherapy For Osteogenic Sarcoma

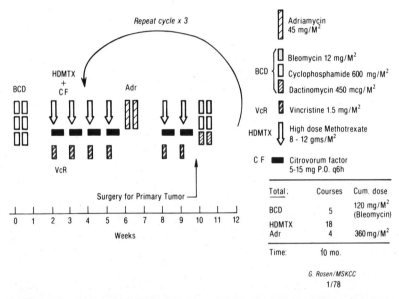

Figure 4 The T-7 protocol used for the treatment of osteosarcoma. Patients receive a combination of bleomycin, cyclophosphamide, and dactinomycin (BCD) for their first course of chemotherapy, and the effect of this treatment on the primary tumor is recorded. Two weeks after BCD they start weekly HDMTX with CFR. The starting dose of HDMTX is 8 gms/m² in adolescents and 12 gms/m² in children below the age of 12 years. The dose of HDMTX is escalated by 2-gm increments if objective evidence of tumor regression dose not occur while the patient is receiving HDMTX with CFR. In most patients a response is observable at a dose between 12 and 16 grams of MTX (total dose). Older patients frequently complain of vincristine-related neurotoxicity (generalized aches and pains), and the vincristine is frequently omitted in such patients. Surgery for the primary tumor is performed at the time indicated or at a later time if a custom-made endoprosthesis is not yet available for patients undergoing en bloc resection and total femur replacement.[7] Postoperative chemotherapy is then continued when good wound healing has been achieved (usually between 2 and 6 weeks following surgery).

some investigators to speculate on the role of this agent in management of untreated patients.[29] The drug usually produces some renal toxicity in the majority of patients given therapeutic doses.[52] It has also been our experience that many patients treated with therapeutic doses plus mannitol for diuresis to prevent renal toxicity develop some impairment of renal function. This may be manifested initially by a marked decrease in the creatinine clearance after two or three courses of treatment and will preclude treatment with MTX-CF. Therefore, it should be used only after resistance to MTX-CF has developed. Such resistance can only be determined if the patient has received sufficient escalation of the MTX dose in excess of 12 gm/m² and still demonstrates progression of disease.

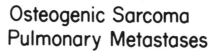

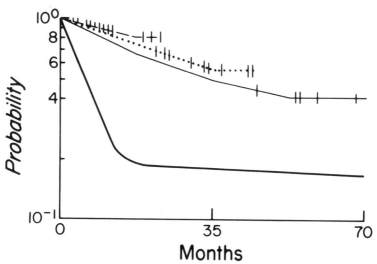

		Free	Relap	Total	Median
——	Study 1	5	7	12	34.4
·······	Study 2	13	9	22	
– – –	Study 3	22	3	25	
——	Historical Controls				

Figure 5 Results of three adjuvant studies utilizing V-MTX-CF and ADR. The results are updated to January 1978. The historical control series represents 78 previously treated patients in whom local control was achieved by amputation.

114

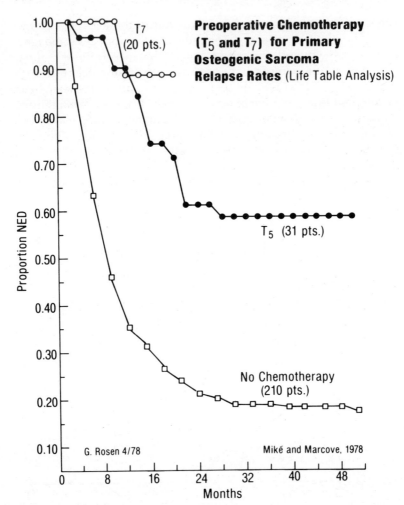

Preoperative Chemotherapy (T5 and T7) for Primary Osteogenic Sarcoma Relapse Rates (Life Table Analysis)

T7 (20 pts.)

T5 (31 pts.)

No Chemotherapy (210 pts.)

G. Rosen 4/78

Miké and Marcove, 1978

Proportion NED

Months

Figure 6 The effect of preoperative chemotherapy in prolonging the disease-free survival in patients with osteosarcoma. The lower curve shows the relapse rate (patients developing pulmonary metastases) of 210 patients who had amputation followed by no chemotherapy. The middle curve shows the disease-free survival of 31 patients treated with "T-5" chemotherapy.[17] These patients received 2 to 3 doses of HDMTX and adriamycin prior to en bloc resection of the primary tumor (distal femur or proximal tibia lesions); 60% of these patients remained completely free of disease. Five of the relapsing patients developed late solitary pulmonary metastases which were resected, and these 5 patients continue to remain free of disease following the additional administration of MTX-CF. Therefore, the overall disease-free survival of patients receiving T-5 chemotherapy is 74%. T-5 chemotherapy initially consisted of only 6 doses of MTX-CF in addition to adriamycin and cyclophosphamide. The top curve represents 20 patients receiving preoperative T-7 chemotherapy (see Figure 4). All patients received preoperative chemotherapy regardless of the site of their primary tumor. Only one patient has relapsed at this early time, and he is currently free of disease following thoracotomy and continued MTX-CF.

Table 1
Chemotherapy for Osteosarcoma

Investigator	Vincristine	Methotrexate (MTX)	Citrovorum factor (CF)	Adriamycin	Cyclophosphamide	L-phenylalanine mustard (L-PAM)	Cis-dichlorodiammine platinum II (DPP)	*Life Table* Disease-free Survival
Eilber et al.[a]	1-5 mg/m²	100-200 mg/kg	12 mg q6h x 72 hrs	45 mg/m² x 2 q2 weeks (max. 500 mg/m²)	—	—	—	60%
Freeman et al.[b]	—	—	—	30 mg/m²/d x 3 (max. 540 mg/m²)			Variable doses, eg. 20 mg/m²/d x 4 120 Mg/m²/d q3-4 wk	—
Jaffe et al.[c]	2 mg/m² (max. 2 mg)	3-7.5 gm/m² 6 hr infusion	15 mg q 3-6h x 72 hrs	75 mg q3h (max. 450 mg/m²)	—	—	—	40-65%
Pratt et al.[d]	—	100-300 mg/kg 6 hr infusion	5 mg/kg over 24 hrs; then 12 mg/m² q6h x 48 hrs	25 mg/m² x 2 q 4 weeks x 10 cycles	600 mg/m²	—	—	—
Rosen et al.[e]	1.5 mg/m² (deleted if patient has vincristine-related toxicity)	8-12 gm/m² 4 hr infusion	10 mg q6h x 10	1.5 mg/kg or 45 mg/m² (max. 360-450 mg/m²)	1200 mg/m² in combination with bleomycin & dactinomycin	—	—	65%-90%

Table 1 *(Continued)*

Investigator	Vincristine	Methotrexate (MTX)	Citrovorum factor (CF)	Adriamycin	Cyclophosphamide	L-phenylalanine mustard (L-PAM)	Cis-dichlorodiammine platinum II (DPP)	*Life Table* Disease-free Survival
Sutow et al.[f]	0.05 mg/kg	75-250 mg/kg 6 hr infusion (3 pulses)	15 mg q3h x 9 followed by 15 mg q6h x 8	Max. 360 mg/m²	10 mg/kg/d x 7 (3 courses)	3 mg/kg x 3 pulses	—	—
							—	—
Wilbur et al.	2 mg/m²	100-300 mg/kg	3-6 mg q3h x 23 doses	60 mg/m² (max. 300 mg/m²)	10 mg/kg/d x 7 (3 courses)	3 mg/kg x 4 pulses	—	—
							—	—

a. Postoperative treatment.
b. Adriamycin Alternated every 3 weeks with DDP 100/mg/m² as adjuvant therapy.
c. Recent programs commence with 7.5 gm/m² q wk x 4.
d. Reduced dose of MTX for "clinically localized" disease.
e. T-4 and T-5 protocol. Current protocol with preoperative chemotherapy given prior to definitive surgery (T-7).
f. COMPADRI-III

CHANGES INDUCED BY CHEMOTHERAPY

Biologic Behavior

The results achieved with effective chemotherapy have produced a number of major changes in the biologic behavior and treatment of osteosarcoma. A reduction in the incidence of pulmonary
metastases has been achieved in the majority of patients. Furthermore, patients who do relapse on adjuvant chemotherapy have been
noted to develop less diffuse disease in the lungs which is delayed in
appearance. This has permitted additional numbers of patients to be
rendered tumor-free by the combined treatment of thoracotomy
and continued chemotherapy. In most instances chemotherapy consists of MTX-CF administered at higher doses.[14][31] Occasionally,
radiation therapy has proved to be a valuable adjunct to MTX-CF in
the treatment of bone disease as well as inoperable pulmonary
disease.[37-39] However, the majority of relapsing patients have
their best chance for salvage with the use of thoracotomy where
possible, and additional systemic chemotherapy (see Chapters
11 and 12).[15][53-55]

Patients who relapse with metastatic disease and who are
presumably resistant to adriamycin and MTX-CF (or patients who
cannot receive more adriamycin because the prior cumulative dose
was close to that which might produce cardiotoxicity) may be
treated with a combination of bleomycin, cyclophosphamide, and
dactinomycin.[56] This combination has been shown to have a
response rate in excess of 60% in patients with evaluable disease.
Because of its efficacy it has been incorporated into the adjuvant
chemotherapy protocol for previously untreated patients (Figure 4).
As indicated earlier, cis-dichlorodiammine platinum (II) has also
been shown to be effective in patients with advanced disease.

Primary Tumor

With the availability of effective chemotherapy, innovative
approaches to the treatment of the primary tumor have been introduced. These include resections and endoprosthetic bone
replacements for tumors of the femur, and modified Tikhoff-Linberg
procedures as previously described by Kotz and Salzer.[57-59] An
Austin-Moore prosthesis to provide an elongated stump capable of
bearing a suction-fitting midthigh prosthesis has been provided for
younger patients with lesions of the distal femur who otherwise
might have had to undergo hip disarticulation and wear a Canadian
bucket prosthesis.[58] "Turn-about" procedures converting the ankle

into a knee have also been performed in such patients. Finally, transmedullary amputation rather than disarticulation has been employed with increasing frequency for lesions of the distal and middle portions of the femur (see Chapters 9 and 10).[60]

The foregoing procedures require the utmost in surgical skill to obtain tumor-free margins. Poor cancer surgery cannot be excused in the hope that effective systemic chemotherapy will prove to be an adequate substitute. The latter may be ineffective against bulk tumor and may mask a local recurrence which may appear long after the cessation of treatment. Chemotherapy is also maximally effective against microscopic disease. It is for this reason that transmedullary amputations are performed at least 7 cm above the most proximal site visible on bone scanning.[60]

The value of preoperative chemotherapy for limb preservation has been documented by several investigators.[17][31][57][61-63] Rosen and Marcove have extended this approach even to include patients undergoing amputation, based on the following assumptions:[31]

1. Early systemic chemotherapy provides immediate treatment for disseminated systemic micrometastases without waiting for the patient to recover from a major surgical procedure.

2. The oncologist has an opportunity to determine the effective dose of MTX-CF in the individual patient. Such treatment can be administered weekly by those familiar with its use.

3. Preoperative chemotherapy provides time for the surgeon to plan limb-salvaging resectional surgery if evaluation of the patient before surgery makes this advisable. In some instances the manufacture of a custom-fitted endoprosthesis is necessary, and this may require 2 to 3 months.

4. If necessary, the dose of MTX can be increased so as to achieve a response in the patient's primary tumor. This will be the correct dose for that individual patient. An assessment of the primary tumor is made at weekly intervals with careful clinical measurements including notation of symptomatic relief, repeated measurements of serum alkaline phosphatase in patients in whom it is elevated, and frequent bone scans (Figure 7).

Utilizing the above principles in a pilot study of over 20 patients, an actuarial, disease-free survival as high as 90% at a follow-up period of approximately 18 months has been achieved (Figure 6). In addition, many patients who received preoperative chemotherapy had appropriate upward adjustments in MTX dosage until regression of the primary tumor was believed to have occurred.

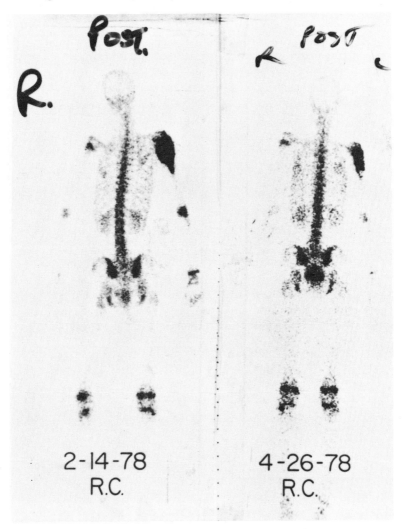

Figure 7 Technetium[99] diphosphonate bone scans of a patient with osteosarcoma of the proximal humerus. These bone scans were done before (left) and during (right) T-7 chemotherapy. Following the first dose of HDMTX, the patient's pain decreased markedly. This led us to believe that she was receiving effective preoperative chemotherapy. The patient also had a lowering of her abnormally elevated serum alkaline phosphatase, and the effect of chemotherapy was confirmed not only by the repeated bone scan but by histologic confirmation of tumor response following *en bloc* resection of the proximal humerus, clavicle, and scapula (Tikhoff-Linberg procedure).

The favorable effects of chemotherapy on the primary tumor were also demonstrated histologically following surgical removal of the primary tumor.[17 51 57 61 63] This was also noted in an analysis of 31 patients who underwent preoperative chemotherapy with MTX-CF and adriamycin prior to limb-salvaging surgery. Most patients had their dosage of MTX increased to achieve a favorable response, but this procedure was not routine in all of the 31 patients. In addition, they received only six doses of MTX-CF for the entire course of chemotherapy (with the addition of adriamycin and cyclophosphamide) because the lack of extensive experience at that time made the administration of MTX-CF more hazardous. Fifteen patients achieved an almost complete response (histologically) of the primary tumor to chemotherapy, and all 15 are still surviving between three and four years from the time of surgery (Figures 8 and 9). In contrast, of 16 patients who had no favorable response to preoperative chemotherapy or only a partial response, only 53% are surviving free of disease between 3 and 4 years from the institution of systemic chemotherapy.[31]

Thus, the rationale of using systemic chemotherapy for all patients with osteosarcoma and, perhaps, other solid tumors also, might evolve to include early preoperative (postbiopsy) chemotherapy while meticulously following each patient to achieve the maximal effect of chemotherapy on the primary tumor. Particularly in the treatment of the malignant spindle cell sarcomas where MTX-CF appears to be effective, the dose of MTX should be

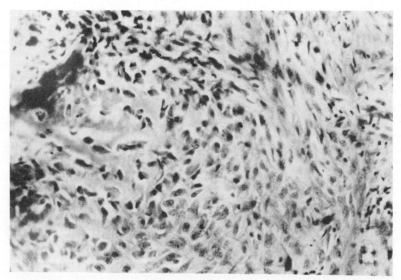

Figure 8 Biopsy of a fully malignant osteosarcoma demonstrating an active spindle cell sarcomatous stroma with areas of abundant osteoid production.

escalated to that required to achieve a response in any given tumor. This would ensure that each patient receives treatment with the maximally effective dose of systemic chemotherapy as defined by the patient, the biologic behavior of the tumor, and his ability to tolerate the maximally effective dose of the drug.

The foregoing recommendations are based on the assumption that chemotherapy will achieve some degree of tumor destruction in all patients. However, tumor destruction may be incomplete and, occasionally, chemotherapy may be ineffective. Under these circumstances preoperative chemotherapy constitutes a delay in tumor eradication, and the risk for the development of pulmonary metastases may be enhanced without surgical intervention. The magnitude of this potential risk is unknown since the destruction of microscopic disease and bulk tumor may be governed by different factors. Until such information is accumulated, it has been decided to perform limb preservation at SFCI-CHMC by means of primary surgical resection. A supply of prefabricated endoprostheses for this purpose has been obtained.

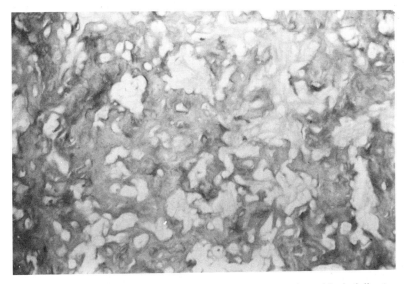

Figure 9 Histologic section of an osteosarcoma removed en block following preoperative T-7 chemotherapy. This section shows abundant tumor osteoid with no evidence of viable tumor cells. The appearance of the tumor demonstrates the effect of chemotherapy on the primary tumor which can be achieved with aggressive preoperative chemotherapy. It is hoped and assumed that systemic micrometastases undergo similar effects while the patient is receiving preoperative chemotherapy. The latter is probably true since retrospective analysis of patients receiving such treatment prior to en bloc resection of the primary tumor (T-5 protocol—see Figure 6) showed that of 15 patients demonstrating an effect of chemotherapy on the primary tumor similar to the above histologic appearance, all 15 are long-term disease-free survivors.[31]

GIANT CELL TUMORS

Giant cell tumors are extremely rare in the pediatric-age group, but occur with increasing frequency in adolescents. These tumors classically arise in the epiphysis of a bone and appear as a localized lytic lesion. They are common in the long bones of the extremities but can occur in other sites such as the spine, pelvis, and even in a finger or metatarsal. The majority are of low-grade malignancy, and local intervention by surgical treatment may be sufficient. Cryosurgery has greatly decreased the local recurrence rate and has allowed more conservative limb-preserving surgery.[64] The addition of this modality to the surgical treatment of giant cell tumors represents a significant advance. In the past a high recurrence rate following curettage alone has been noted. Giant cell tumors in the spine or pelvis present a particularly difficult situation because, although they may be benign histologically, they can produce severe debility and even death. In this situation, radiation therapy may be attempted to try to control the surgically unapproachable tumor; however, radiation therapy has been associated with malignant transformation of giant cell tumors in the past.[65] A fully malignant giant cell tumor may be encountered occasionally in which the sarcomatous stroma resembles that of a fully malignant spindle cell sarcoma. In such cases systemic chemotherapy may be utilized in an attempt to prevent the occurrence of distant metastases. Occasionally, even what is called a low-grade benign giant cell tumor has been noted to produce pulmonary metastases.[66]

CHONDROSARCOMA, FIBROSARCOMA, AND OTHER SPINDLE CELL SARCOMAS

These spindle cell sarcomas may be encountered in children and adolescents. In the general population, the majority are of low-grade malignancy. An experienced pathologist should have available all of the clinical material such as a roentgenogram and the age of the patient prior to review of the biopsy, since tumors that appear malignant in early childhood and infancy may have benign courses. An example is juvenile fibromatosis, which should be treated by local excision without systemic chemotherapy. This rarely represents a metastasizing tumor.[67]

Most chondrosarcomas or fibrosarcomas of bone in adolescents have a high grade of malignancy and tend to metastasize; therefore, most patients will require systemic chemotherapy. The chemotherapy utilized for this group of diseases is similar to that used in the treatment of osteosarcoma. In our experience, although rare in childhood, three of four patients presenting with pure, high-grade, fully malignant chondrosarcomas have responded favorably to treatment with MTX-CF. These patients were subsequently placed on a protocol similar to that used for the treatment of osteosarcoma. Such treatment for malignant chondrosarcomas appears to be effective. However, in treating patients with primarily chondroblastic osteosarcoma, one of us (G.R.) has noted the chondrosarcomatous component is slightly more resistant than either the fibroblastic or osteogenic areas. Therefore, in treating fully malignant chondrosarcoma, an attempt is made to try to escalate the dose of MTX to the maximal tolerated level, or one which gives a demonstrable effect of the chemotherapy on the primary tumor.[17]

Of the other malignant spindle cell sarcomas of bone and soft tissue, the entity known as malignant fibrous histiocytoma of both bone and soft tissue is being diagnosed with greater frequency since the initial description of these pathologic entities.[68][69] These tumors are spindle cell sarcomas that have a fibrous stroma. The majority of these in children and adolescents are fully malignant. They derive their name from the fact that histiocytes can be seen along with the malignant spindle cells, and it is the opinion of most pathologists that this malignant tumor has a histiocytic origin. Patients with fully malignant fibrous histiocytoma of soft tissue, or of bone treated with ablative surgery alone, have approximately a 60% to 70% chance of developing systemic metastases following treatment. Therefore, it has been our policy to treat all of these patients with systemic therapy.

In the past 12 patients with spindle cell sarcomas such as fully malignant fibrosarcoma, malignant fibrous histiocytoma, and synovial sarcomas of the soft tissue have received adjuvant chemotherapy following surgery at MSKCC, and all have remained free of metastatic disease for a follow-up period of up to 4 years. Without adjuvant chemotherapy, approximately two thirds of these patients would have been expected to develop metastases. The agents utilized for systemic chemotherapy for this group of patients were similar to those used for osteosarcoma, but MTX-CF was given less often since these tumors do not metastasize as rapidly as osteosarcoma nor are they as resistant as chondrosarcoma. Regression of metastatic tumor has been observed not only with MTX-CF but also with cyclophosphamide, adriamycin, and the combination of bleomycin, cyclophosphamide, and dactinomycin.

CHEMOTHERAPY-RELATED CONSIDERATIONS

MTX is excreted primarily by the kidneys. Consequently, a

creatinine clearance must be performed prior to its administration. Additional biochemical evaluations for monitoring toxicity include liver function studies, since many of the cytotoxic agents, including high-dose MTX, are potentially hepatotoxic. It should be noted that following MTX-CF, there is usually a transient increase in the SGOT. However, in the majority of patients liver function studies become normal within one to two weeks. Not infrequently, the serum alkaline phosphatase will be elevated as a reflection of tumor activity in patients with osteosarcoma. In such instances it is necessary to determine the serum level of 5′ nucleotidase to assist in the evaluation of liver function. The serum alkaline phosphatase can be used only as a "tumor marker" in patients who have normal liver function tests including SGOT and 5′ nucleotidase.

Following MTX-CF patients should be observed daily for at least 3 to 4 days. Indications for additional intravenous hydration include: 1) An abnormally elevated serum MTX level on any of the three days following administration of MTX-CF. 2) An early rise in the serum creatinine in the first one to three days following the administration of MTX-CF. 3) A decrease in the daily weight (300 gm) following administration of MTX-CF. 4) The failure to maintain an adequately alkaline urine. Most patients at MSKCC are expected to excrete a minimum of 2000 ml/m²/24 hours of alkaline urine. Failure to do so on follow-up examination in one of the three days following MTX is an indication for additional intravenous hydration and/or intravenous bicarbonate to insure an alkaline urine. 5) In addition, the early development of clinical manifestations of drug toxicity, including stomatitis with consequent difficulty in obtaining a high oral intake of fluids, or early leukopenia is an indication for additional intravenous hydration of the patient in the first few days following MTX-CF.[18]

Patients who present with very bulky tumors or pleural effusions may be expected to have a late release of MTX from this "third space," and continued monitoring of serum MTX levels may be necessary in such patients.[21] CF probably does not "rescue" a patient until at least 48 hours following the administration of MTX-CF. This is because CF has to compete with MTX for entry into the normal cell. Thus, if serum MTX levels are abnormally high, particularly after 48 hours following the administration of MTX-CF, higher doses of CF than are conventionally used to help "rescue" the patient and prevent toxicity may be indicated.[70] However, the assurance of good renal clearance of MTX early in the course following MTX-CF is probably the best way to prevent drug-related toxicity.

It has been our experience that the majority of the side effects usually observed after treatment with high doses of MTX-CF are reversible and do not produce permanent damage, however. The recommendation for treatment with chemotherapy carries a commitment that it will be administered under expert supervision. This should include facilities where measures to prevent and treat toxicity are immediately available.

REFERENCES

1. Ahiua, S.C., Villacin, A.B., Smith, J., et al: Juxtacortical (parosteal) osteogenic sarcoma. *J Bone Joint Surg* [Am] 59A:632–647, 1977.

2. Burchenal, J.H.: From wild fowl to stalking horses: Alchemy of chemotherapy. Fifth Annual D.A. Karnofsky Memorial Lecture. *Cancer* 35:1121–1135, 1975.

3. Skipper, H.E., Schabel, F.M., Jr., and Wilcox, W.S.: Experimental evaluation of potential anticancer agents—XIII. On the criteria and kinetics associated with "curability" of experimental leukemia. *Cancer Chemother Rep* 35:1–111, 1964.

4. Skipper, H.E., Schabel, F.M., Jr., and Wilcox, W.S.: Experimental evaluation of potential anticancer agents—XIV. Further study of certain basic concepts underlying chemotherapy of leukemia. *Cancer Chemother Rep* 45:5–28, 1965.

5. Laster, W.R., Jr., Mayo, J.G., Simpson-Herren, L., et al: Success and failure in the treatment of solid tumors-II. Kinetic parameters and "cell cure" of moderately advanced carcinoma 755. *Cancer Chemother Rep* 53:169–188, 1969.

6. Pinkel, D.: Five year follow-up of "total therapy" of childhood lymphocytic leukemia. *JAMA* 216:648–652, 1971.

7. Holland, J.F. and Glidewell, O.: Oncologists' reply: Survival expectancy in acute lymphocytic leukemia, editorial. *N Engl Med* 287:769–777, 1972.

8. DeVita, V.T., Jr., Chabner, B., Hubbard, S.P., et al: Advanced diffuse histiocytic lymphoma, a potentially curable disease. *Lancet* 1:248–250, 1975.

9. Farber, S.: Chemotherapy in the treatment of leukemia and Wilms' tumor. *JAMA* 198:826–836, 1969.

10. Schabel, F.M., Jr.: Concepts for systemic treatment of micrometastases. *Cancer* 35:15–24, 1975.

11. Jaffe, N., Farber, S., Traggis, D., et al: Favorable response of osteogenic sarcoma to high dose methotrexate with citrovorum rescue and radiation therapy. *Cancer* 31:1367–1373, 1973.

12. Jaffe, N.: Recent advances in the chemotherapy of metastatic osteogenic sarcoma. *Cancer* 30:1627–1631, 1972.

13. Fyfe, M.J. and Goldman, I.D.: Characteristics of the

vincristine-induced augmentation of methotrexate uptake in Ehrlich ascites tumor cells. *J Biol Chem* 248:5067–5073, 1973.

14. Rosen, G., Huvos, A.G., Mosende, C., et al: Chemotherapy and thoracotomy for metastatic osteogenic sarcoma: A model for adjuvant chemotherapy and the rationale for the timing of thoracic surgery. *Cancer* 41:841–849, 1978.

15. Rosen, G., Tefft, M., Martinez, A., et al: Combination chemotherapy and radiation therapy in the treatment of metastatic osteogenic sarcoma. *Cancer* 35:622–630, 1975.

16. Beattie, E.J., Jr., Martini, N., and Rosen, G.: The management of pulmonary metastases in children with osteogenic sarcoma with surgical resection combined with chemotherapy. *Cancer* 35:618–621, 1975.

17. Rosen, G., Murphy, M.L., Huvos, A.G., et al: Chemotherapy, *en bloc* resection, and prosthetic bone replacement in the treatment of osteogenic sarcoma. *Cancer* 37:1–11, 1976.

18. Nirenberg, A., Mosende, C., Rosen, G., et al: High dose methotrexate with citrovorum factor rescue: Predictive value of serum methotrexate concentrations and corrective measures to avert toxicity. *Cancer Treat Rep* 61:779–783, 1977.

19. Chan, H., Evans, W.E., and Pratt, C.G.: Recovery from toxicity associated with high dose methotrexate: Prognosis factors. *Cancer Treat Rep* 61:797–804, 1977.

20. Etcubanas, E. and Wilbur, J.R.: Adjuvant chemotherapy for osteogenic sarcoma. *Cancer Treat Rep* 62:283–287, 1978.

21. Jaffe, N. and Traggis, D.: Toxicity of high dose methotrexate (NSC-740) and citrovorum factor (NSC-3590) in osteogenic sarcoma. *Cancer Chemother Rep* 6:31–36, 1975.

22. Cortes, E.P., Holland, J.F., Wang, J.J., et al: Chemotherapy of advanced osteosarcoma. Reprinted from Vol. 24 of the Colston Papers, *Proceedings of the 24th Symposium of the Colston Research Society.* London, Butterworth, 1972.

23. Cortes, E.P., Holland, J.F., Wang, J.J., et al: Amputation and adriamycin in primary osteosarcoma. *N Engl J Med* 291:998–1000, 1974.

24. Sullivan, M.P., Sutow, W.W., and Taylor, G.: L-phenylalanine mustard as a treatment for metastatic osteogenic sarcoma in children. *J Pediatr* 63:227, 1963.

25. Evans, A.E., Heyn, R., Nesbit, M., et al: Evaluation of mitomycin-C (NSC-26980) in the treatment of metastatic osteogenic sarcoma. *Cancer Chemother Rep* 53:297, 1969.

26. Sutow, W.W.: Evaluation of dosage schedules of mitomycin-C (NSC-26980) in children. *Cancer Chemother Rep* 55:285, 1971.

27. Pinkel, D.: Cyclophosphamide in children with cancer. *Cancer* 15:42–49, 1969.

28. Pratt, C.B., Hustu, H.O., and Shanks, E.: Cyclic multiple drug adjuvant chemotherapy for osteosarcoma. *Proc AACR/ASCO** 15:19, 1974.

29. Ochs, J.J., Freeman, A.I., Douglas, H.O., Jr., et al: Cis-dichlorodiammine-platinum (II) in advanced osteogenic sarcoma. *Cancer Treat Rep* 62:239–245, 1978.

30. Rosen, G.: The development of an adjuvant chemotherapy program for the treatment of osteogenic sarcoma. *Front Rad Ther Oncol* 10:115–133, 1975.

31. Rosen, G., Marcove, R.C., Caparros, B., et al: Primary osteogenic sarcoma: The rationale for preoperative chemotherapy and delayed surgery. Submitted for publication.

32. Jaffe, N., Frei, E., III, Traggis, D., et al: Adjuvant methotrexate-citrovorum factor of osteogenic sarcoma. *N Engl J Med* 291:994–997, 1974.

33. Marcove, R.C., Mike, V., Hajek, J.V., et al: Osteogenic sarcoma under the age of twenty-one. A review of one hundred and forty-five operative cases. *J Bone Joint Surg* [Am] 55:411–423, 1970.

34. Jaffe, N.: The potential for an improved prognosis with chemotherapy in osteogenic sarcoma. *Clin Orthop* 113:111–118, 1975.

35. Jaffe, N.: Osteogenic sarcoma — State of the art with high dose methotrexate treatment. *Clin Orthop* 120:95–102, 1976.

36. Jaffe, N. and Frei, E., III: Osteogenic sarcoma: Advances in treatment. *CA* 26:351–359, 1976.

37. Jaffe, N., Traggis, D., Cassady, J.R., et al: Advances in the treatment of osteogenic sarcoma, in Tagnon, H.J. and Staquet, M.J. (eds): *Recent Advances in Cancer Treatment*. New York, Raven Press, 1977.

38. Jaffe, N., Frei, E., III, Watts, H., et al: High dose methotrexate in osteogenic sarcoma: A 5-year experience. *Cancer Treat Rep* 62:259–264, 1978.

39. Jaffe, N., Traggis, D., Cassady, J.R., et al: The role of high dose methotrexate with citrovorum factor "rescue" in the treatment of osteogenic sarcoma. *Int J Radiat Biol* 2:261–266, 1977.

40. Rosen, G., Suwansirikul, S., Kwon, C., et al: High dose methotrexate with citrovorum factor rescue and adriamycin in childhood osteogenic sarcoma. *Cancer* 33:1151–1163, 1974.

41. Rosen, G., Tan, C., Exelby, P., et al: Vincristine, high dose methotrexate with citrovorum factor rescue, cyclophosphamide and adriamycin cyclic therapy following surgery in childhood osteogenic sarcoma. *Proc AACR/ASCO** 15:172, 1974.

42. Rosen, G., Tan, C., Sanmaneechai, A., et al: The rationale for multiple drug chemotherapy in the treatment of osteogenic sarcoma. *Cancer* 35:936–945, 1975.

43. Sutow, W.W., Sullivan, M.P., Fernbach, et al: Adjuvant chemotherapy in primary treatment of osteogenic sarcoma. A Southwest Oncology Group Study. *Cancer* 36:1598–1602, 1975.

44. Sutow, W.W., Gehan, E.A., Vietti, T.J., et al: Multidrug chemotherapy in primary treatment of osteosarcoma. *J Bone Joint Surg.* [Am] 58A:629–633, 1976.

45. Sutow, W.W., Gehan, E.A., Dyment, P.G., et al: Multidrug adjuvant chemotherapy for osteosarcoma: Interim report of the Southwest Oncology Group Studies. *Cancer Treat Rep* 62:265–269, 1978.

46. Eilber, F.R., Grant, T., and Morton, D.L.: Adjuvant therapy for osteosarcoma: Preoperative and postoperative treatment. *Cancer Treat Rep* 62:213–216, 1978.

47. Ettinger, L.J., Douglass, H.O., Jr., Higby, D.J., et al: Adjuvant adriamycin (ADR) and cis-diammine dichloroplatinum (DDP) in primary osteogenic sarcoma. *Proc AACR/ASCO** 19:323, 1978.

48. Pratt, C.B., Rivera, G., Shanks, E., et al: Combination chemotherapy for osteosarcoma. *Cancer Treat Rep* 62:251–257, 1978.

49. Carter, S.K. and Friedman, M.: Osteogenic sarcoma treatment overview and some comments on interpretation of clinical trial data. *Cancer Treat Rep* 62:199–204, 1978.

50. Shepp, M., Necheles, T.F., Banks, H.H., et al: Adjuvant treatment of osteogenic sarcoma with high dose cyclophosphamide. *Cancer Teat Rep.* 62:295–296, 1978.

51. Huvos, A., Rosen, G., and Marcove, R.C.: Primary osteogenic sarcoma: Pathologic aspects in 20 patients after treatment with chemotherapy, *en bloc* resection, and prosthetic bone replacement. *Arch Pathol Lab Med* 101:14–18, 1977.

52. Dentino, M., Luft, F.C., Yum, M.N., et al: Long-term effect of cis-diamminedichloride platinum (CDDP) on renal function and structure in man. *Cancer* 41:1274–1281, 1978.

53. Jaffe, N., Traggis, D., Cassady, J.R., et al: Multidisciplinary treatment for macrometastatic osteogenic sarcoma. *Br Med J* 2:1039–1041, 1976.

54. Jaffe, N.: Progress report on high dose methotrexate (NSC-740) with citrovorum factor rescue in the treatment of metastatic bone tumor. *Cancer Chemother Rep* 58:275–280, 1974.

---

*AACR/ASCO — American Association for Cancer Research/American Society of Clinical Oncology.

55. Jaffe, N., Frei, E., III, Traggis, D., et al: High dose methotrexate with citrovorum factor in osteogenic sarcoma — Progress Report II. *Cancer Treat Rep* 61:675-679, 1977.

56. Mosende, C., Caparros, B., Rosen, G., et al: Combination chemotherapy with bleomycin, cyclophosphamide and dactinomycin for the treatment of osteogenic sarcoma. *Cancer* 40:2779-2786, 1977.

57. Jaffe, N., Frei, E., III, Traggis, D., et al: Weekly high dose methotrexate-citrovorum factor in osteogenic sarcoma: Pre-surgical treatment of primary tumor and of overt pulmonary metastases. *Cancer* 39:45-50, 1977.

58. Rosen, G.: Malignant bone tumors: Current management. *Pediatr Ann* in press.

59. Kotz, R. and Salzer, M.: Resection therapy of malignant tumors of the shoulder girdle. *Osterreichische Zeitschrift für Onkologie* 2:97-109, 1975.

60. Jaffe, N. and Watts, H.: Multidrug chemotherapy in primary treatment of osteosarcoma. *J Bone Joint Surg* [Am] 58A:5:634-635, 1976.

61. Jaffe, N., Watts, H., Fellows, K.E., et al: Local *en bloc* resection for limb preservation. *Cancer Treat Rep* 62:217-223, 1978.

62. Jaffe, N., Watts, H., Frei, E., et al: Limb preservation in osteogenic sarcoma: A preliminary report in Tagon, H.J. and Staquet, M.J. (eds): *Recent Advances in Cancer Treatment*. New York, Raven Press, 1977, pp 114-220.

63. Morton, D.L., Eilber, F.R., Townsend, C.M., Jr., et al: Limb salvage from a multidisciplinary treatment approach for skeletal and soft tissue sarcomas of the extremity. *Ann Surg* 184:268-278, 1976.

64. Marcove, R.C., Weis, L.D., Vaghaiwalla, M.R., et al: Cryosurgery in the treatment of giant cell tumors of bone: A report of 52 consecutive cases. *Cancer* 41:957-969, 1978.

65. Spjut, H.J., Dorman, H.D., Fechner, R.E., et al: Tumors of Uncertain Origin, in *Tumors of Bone and Cartilage*. Washington, Armed Forces Institute of Pathology, US Government Printing Office, 1970, pp 293-315.

66. Jewell, J.H. and Bush, L.F.: Benign giant cell tumors of bone with a solitary pulmonary metastasis: A case report. *J Bone Joint Surg* [Am] 46:A:848-852, 1964.

67. Stout, A.P.: Juvenile fibromatosis. *Cancer* 7:953, 1954.

68. Dahlin, D.C., Unni, K.K., and Matsuno, T.: Malignant fibrous histiocytoma of bone — Fact or fancy. *Cancer* 39:508, 1977.

69. Huvos, A.G.: Primary malignant fibrous histiocytoma of bone. Clinicopathologic study of 18 patients. *NY State J Med* 76:552, 1976.

70. Isacoff, W.H., Aroesty, J., Willis, K.L., et al: Pharmacokinetics of high dose methotrexate with citrovorum factor rescue. *Cancer Treat Rep* 61:(Part II) 1665, 1977.

8 Surgical Management of Malignant Bone Tumors in Children

Hugh G. Watts, M.D.

Prior to the advent of chemotherapy, the treatment of osteosarcomas was wholly within the surgeon's purview. Amputation was the usual treatment, and any debate focused on the level of the amputation. The introduction of complex regimens of chemotherapy led to the intimidation of the surgeon, leaving him on the periphery playing the role of ablating technician. If the patient is to receive the best therapy, this should not be the case. The biopsy must be done properly and the surgical options known. The effects of chemotherapy on surgery and postsurgical rehabilitation also must be understood.

BIOPSY

The biopsy of potentially malignant bone tumors should be as much a part of the overall planning for the patient as any subsequent surgery. If an amputation is anticipated, the biopsy must be performed at a site which will not interfere with the amputation flaps.

131

Recent changes in treatment allow for resection of some osteosarcomas without amputation. In such situations the location of the biopsy is critical, since the site must be removed en bloc with the tumor. If the biopsy site is to be excised with the tumor, it is preferable to obtain the sample with a minimum of traction and dissection. For example, the customary technique for obtaining a biopsy specimen from the distal femur is to retract the vastus, medialis, or lateralis anteriorly. However, if this approach is used, subsequent excision of the extensively contaminated biopsy tract may lead to wound closure difficulties, as well as decreased postoperative function.

Tumors of the proximal tibia are more readily resected with a medial approach, and therefore the biopsy site should be on the medial side. Classically, however, a proximal tibial biopsy is performed through an oblique incision in line with the pes anserinus, and this presents difficulties for the surgeon performing the subsequent resection since his incision, ordinarily a longitudinal one, will be at right angles to the line of the biopsy incision.

The possibility of radiation treatment should be considered when planning the biopsy. Pathologic fracture of an irradiated bone is a frequent problem, especially when chemotherapy is superimposed. If a tumor appears to be potentially radioresponsive, the surgeon should attempt to obtain a sample of tumor outside of the bone without violating the cortex. If the cortex of the bone must be invaded, the cortical hole should not be a "window" but a "porthole." A rectangle with sharp corners provides four areas of stress-concentration, resulting in an increased possibility of pathologic fracture. The porthole should be as small as possible yet provide an adequate specimen for diagnosis.

If radiation treatment is anticipated, the radiation therapist should be consulted before the biopsy is done. He must include the biopsy site in the radiation field yet allow a strip of nonirradiated skin for lymphatic drainage of the distal segment. For example, if radiation of a femoral lesion has to include the inguinal nodes and iliac vessels, it is preferable to biopsy the tumor from the medial rather than the lateral side if possible.

Primary bone malignancies are often histologically heterogeneous. Needle biopsies do not usually provide satisfactory specimens. The consequences of misdiagnosis are enormous, and needle biopsy is best reserved for areas which are difficult to reach, such as vertebral bodies, or for confirming that a second skeletal lesion contains tumor cells.

Those not accustomed to dealing with skeletal tumors frequently find it necessary to do a second biopsy to obtain adequate tissue. To prevent this, it is advisable to obtain a frozen section of the biopsy specimen to establish that it is adequate for making a diagnosis when the tissue is finally prepared.

There are many types of tumors which can involve bone in children. Management falls roughly into two categories: (a) those treated primarily by surgery with or without chemotherapy (eg, osteosarcoma); and (2) those treated primarily by radiation and chemotherapy (eg, Ewing's sarcoma). Osteosarcoma and Ewing's sarcoma will be discussed separately and in detail. The principles outlined for these prototypes can be followed for the management of the less common tumors.

OSTEOSARCOMA

Amputation

Except with parosteal lesions, amputation is still the treatment of choice for primary osteosarcoma. However, the introduction of use of massive doses of toxic chemotherapeutic agents has altered the surgeon's management.

Timing Amputation of an extremity immediately following biopsy and frozen section has not lead to any increase in survival.[1] Diagnosis of bone tumors by frozen section can be treacherous. In a child, operative procedure and postoperative care will proceed more smoothly if there is adequate time for emotional preparation for an amputation. A delay of several days after biopsy will not affect patient survival, and the child and parents can be told that amputation definitely is needed.[2] This will allow a suitable interval in which to prepare the child through discussion of problems he will encounter after amputation—such as phantom limb sensation and limits on his range of activities. Preamputation instruction in walking with crutches can be given, and where possible the child can meet with other amputees who have received similar treatment.

The interval between biopsy and definitive surgery also allows time to explore other options—such as resection—and to make adequate preparations. From a practical point of view, for the surgeon and the operating room personnel, the separation of the biopsy from the amputation permits better organization in scheduling.

Level The appropriate level of amputation in osteosarcoma has always been a point of debate. Should the surgeon remove the entire bone, or should he cut across the bone at some level above the tumor? Surgeons who recommend whole-bone removal cite a local recurrence rate of as high as 21% with transosseous amputations, implying that primary tumor has been left behind.[3] Those who recommend transosseous amputations report a local recurrence rate of less than 5% and blame inappropriate surgical technique for the higher rate cited by others.[4-6]

Distal femoral lesions account for 60% of all osteosarcomas. Surgeons will be faced frequently with the choice of an above-knee amputation with its functional and aesthetic advantages, and a hip disarticulation, which eliminates a fear of leaving tumor behind.

Enneking has documented clinically undetectable intramedullary foci of tumor separate from the primary lesion (so called "skip" lesions), whose existence previously has been questioned.[7] He concludes that cross-bone amputations carry an unacceptably high risk of leaving tumor behind. However, we have adopted a treatment policy of cross-bone amputation and have had no local recurrences (Table 1). Whether these results represent a careful selection of the level at which the bone is transected or the efficacy of chemotherapeutic drugs in eliminating "skip" lesions cannot be stated. At the present time there are no data to demonstrate that survival is enhanced by removing the entire bone.

Table 1
Amputation for Childhood Osteosarcoma

| | Level of Amputation | |
Site	Whole Bone	Transmedullary
Humerus	3(3)*	---
Femur		
Proximal	2(1)	---
Distal	---	32(12)
Tibia		
Proximal	15(4)	---
Distal	---	2(0)
Fibula	1(1)	---
Radius	1	---
Total	22(9)	34(12)
Mean follow-up time	27 mo	38 mo

*Number in parentheses = number of patients who developed metastases. There have been no local recurrences of tumor in patients with transmedullary amputations.

Where should the bone be transected if transosseous amputations are done? Some surgeons will remove the bone as high as the lesser trochanter for a distal femoral lesion. Dahlin and Coventry have demonstrated that transosseous amputation three inches proximal to the tumor as it is seen on plain radiographs can safely remove the tumor. We have a number of cases, though, where tumor extended beyond the limits defined by plain radiographs but could be seen by bone scan. Initially these extensions of increased radionuclide uptake were interpreted as adjacent areas of reactive normal bone. To avoid the possibility of leaving residual tumor, we use the bone scan to help determine the level of bone removal.

A drop of radionuclide—diphosphanate labeled with technetium 99—is placed at one end of a tube (usually the needle cap of a tuberculin syringe). The surgeon places this radioactive pointer on the skin of the affected limb. This will show up as a bright dot on the oscilloscope. The marker is moved proximally or distally on the extremity until the dot is at the level of the most proximal margin of increased radioactive uptake. A polaroid photograph of the oscilloscope is then taken to confirm the location of the radioactive pointer, and the skin is marked with an indelible pen. At the time of amputation a threaded Kirschner wire is inserted into the bone 7.0 cm proximal to the skin mark, and transection is carried out at the level of the wire. Postoperative curettage of the marrow is always performed, but tumor has never been found when the above technique has been used.

Selecting the level of amputation with this technique has resulted in longer stumps compared to levels chosen by less painstaking estimation.

Technique　The standard techniques of amputation must be altered somewhat for patients who will be receiving postoperative chemotherapy. High-dose methotrexate produces some inhibition of healing of the skin, considerable inhibition of healing of the fascia and soft tissues, and marked inhibition of healing of bone. Laboratory examination of the collagen extracted from the skin, fascia, and bone of patients who have had high-dose methotrexate treatment demonstrates marked alteration in the cross-links.

Almost invariably there has been marked soft tissue retraction following amputation when methotrexate has been used. Retraction can be great enough to allow protrusion of the underlying bone through muscle and fascia to the subcutaneous layer. (This is not due to bony overgrowth, a common phenomenon following amputation in children.) Soft tissue retraction is decreased if nonabsorbable sutures are used in attaching the muscles to each other, or to the bone, as well as in the subcutaneous tissues. Skin sutures are best left in place for at least three weeks.

Chemotherapy　We arbitrarily commence chemotherapy with high-dose methotrexate and citrovorum factor "rescue" two weeks after amputation. Initially we started chemotherapy in the recovery room. With this regimen, though, two patients had generalized seizures and there was a greater incidence of drug toxicity, especially in patients undergoing lower extremity amputations, where there is a great deal of postoperative edema. A possible explanation for this phenomenon is that methotrexate is a small molecular weight substance readily able to enter into the edema space, while citrovorum factor is not. Following the "rescue" and discontinuation of citrovorum factor, the methotrexate can leak back from the edema space.

Postoperative management All patients are fitted with plaster dressings and "immediate" postsurgical prostheses. The patients are usually able to walk within two to four days and are discharged within seven to ten days, so they have several days at home before commencing chemotherapy.

The use of high-dose methotrexate alters the stump volume and causes a temporary increase in size during each course of chemotherapy. This must be taken into consideration in prosthetic fitting. The use of a suction socket as the only suspension is unwise. It is preferable to use an auxiliary Silesian belt, which may be discontinued at the end of chemotherapy. To accommodate the frequent changes in stump size caused by chemotherapy we have used a polypropylene "intermediate" prosthesis, which is split medially and laterally to allow an adjustable socket fit (Figure 1). This "intermediate" socket is attached to the "final" endoskeletal limb and is worn for several months after the completion of chemotherapy. The socket is then changed to the "final" one.

Any irritation of the skin from the prosthesis can be frighteningly exaggerated by the use of chemotherapeutic agents, and extra care should be taken to avoid injury with the prosthesis. Our intermediate prostheses are made with a closed-cell polyethylene foam liner to reduce skin irritation.

Postoperative infection in stumps occurred in two patients following amputation. Their chemotherapy was begun on schedule (two weeks postamputation) and the infections were treated by open debridement and closure of the stumps over irrigation tubes. Both amputation stumps healed satisfactorily despite continued administration of chemotherapy.

As a result of the success of chemotherapy, the number of children who are surviving their malignant bone tumors has increased enormously. Children can no longer be relegated to a "wait-and-see" category as regards rehabilitation. They particularly thrive on the athletic programs available to amputees, and participation should be encouraged.

Resection

The new interest in osteosarcoma stimulated by the use of chemotherapy has led to limb-sparing resections of these tumors in a

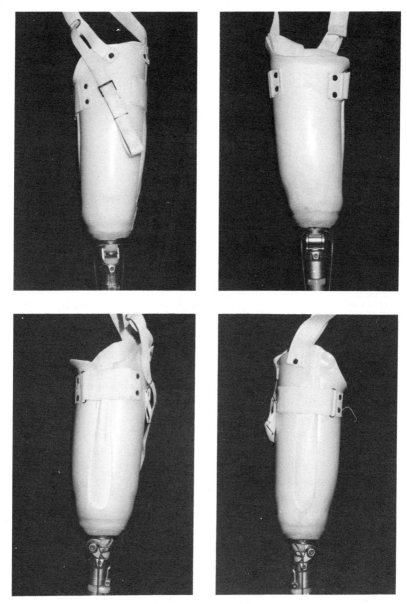

Figure 1. "Intermediate" prosthesis: anterior (**A**), posterior (**B**), medial (**C**), and lateral (**D**) views.

few centers. This is both exciting and potentially hazardous. Can an osteosarcoma be resected without jeopardizing survival? The answer at this time appears to be "yes," *provided an adequate cancer operation is performed.* Our experience is summarized in Table 2.

Table 2
En Block Resection of the Primary Tumor
in Childhood Osteosarcoma

Location	No. of Patients	Subsequent Metastatic Disease	Local Recurrence
Humerus	2	0	0
Femur			
Proximal	1	1*	0
Distal	15	5	1†
Tibia			
Proximal	5	1	0
Midshaft	1	0	0
Fibula	2	0	0
Total	26	7	1

NOTE: Patients aged 10 to 19; follow-up 4 to 42 months (median: 18 months).
* = multifocal disease.
†Tumor cut into at time of resection.

Chemotherapy clearly cannot make up for an inadequate operation. During our first resection, tumor was transected at an area which appeared normal on plain radiograph but which was "hot" by bone scan. Frozen section of the tissue demonstrated tumor. Additional bone was resected at the time of initial surgery. High-dose methotrexate plus Adriamycin did not prevent a local recurrence at the site where the tumor had been entered. Since that time, we have found that resection of 7.0 cm of normal bone proximal or distal to an osteosarcoma as seen by bone scan has proven safe. While a great deal of attention has been focused on the extent of bone proximal to the lesion that must be removed, it must be emphasized that normal tissue around the circumference of the tumor must be excised with it as well.

Vessels are dissected away from the tumor area and held with vascular clips. In distal femoral and proximal tibial lesions this is facilitated if the intervening head of the gastrocnemius muscle is transected early to expose the vessels in an uninvolved area. The gastrocnemius head should not be divided so far distally that its vessels are damaged, since a gastrocnemius muscle flap rotated on its vascular pedicle can be a very useful means of providing soft tissue coverage after resection. In only one case of a fibular osteosarcoma was it necessary to replace the artery (using a saphenous vein graft) at the time of the resection.

Distal femoral tumors frequently erode the knee joint anteriorly, where the suprapatellar pouch extends well above the patella. The absence of tumor cells in joint aspirate does not necessarily rule out invasion of the joint. Therefore, the entire joint—including the patella, the collateral ligaments, and 1.0 to 2.0 cm of the proximal tibia—should be excised.

Once the tumor is resected, the obvious problem is that of reconstructing the colossal defect. There are a number of approaches to reconstruction. In distal femoral lesions, most surgeons have used techniques which allow knee flexion. This has been done using an articulated metallic implant, preferably with intrinsic stability (ie, a joint which can bear full body weight without requiring any active muscle power to maintain knee extension). The use of a metallic implant allows earlier mobilization but requires the use of methylmethacrylate cement to hold the prosthesis in place. The long-term consequences of using cement are not known. Such prostheses with metal-to-metal articulations will become worn and their longevity is not known. Since the excision of the tumor includes the entire joint together with the articulating ligaments, metallic prostheses of only the femur or only the tibia have not been used.

In distal femoral resections, the hamstring muscles may need to be transferred anteriorly to the knee and attached to the infrapatellar ligament to provide active knee extension. This also provides soft tissue cover over the metallic implant.

There is realistic concern about the ability of the metallic implants to withstand the abuse of teenage or young adult activities. For this reason there has been interest in the use of joint allografts, which might provide better long-term results. However, these allografts replace only one side of the joint and retain the host ligaments for joint stability, which violates a potentially tumor-contaminated joint. Also, joint allografts take several years to become incorporated and thus require prolonged protection of the limb. This period will be lengthened by the use of chemotherapy. These years may be the greater part of active childhood, and this is a particular problem for a group of children whose longevity is so unpredictable.

In lesions of the proximal humerus, the tumor is excised, together with the scapula, by a modified Tikhoff-Linberg technique. The humerus is transected 7 cm distal to the lesion as seen by bone scan. The defect is reconstructed by the insertion of a segment of Küntscher rod into the residual humerus. The proximal end of the rod is fixed to the residual clavicle. Initially a small total shoulder unit was used. Subsequently it has been easier to use a piece of a Dacron arterial graft, which is threaded through the extraction hole of the rod and then passed through a hole in the clavicular stump.

Skin sutures are left in for at least one or two months, and chemotherapy is delayed until three weeks after resection. Healing has been a considerable problem. There is a very large skin flap in the resected area and very little soft tissue between the metallic implant and the skin. In our series, three of the ten patients who had resections early in the series eroded the skin through to the metal implant. Two required amputation. Another eroded the skin through an area of previous slough from intra-arterial Adriamycin.

Some surgeons have used radiation to the tumor prior to resection to reduce the possibility of local recurrence. Since the usual doses of radiation are not tumoricidal for osteosarcomas and cannot be relied upon to destroy residual tumor, we feel the problems of wound-healing outweigh any theoretic advantages, and we do not irradiate the areas prior to resection.

Can an osteosarcoma be safely resected and leave a functionally worthwhile limb? Here the answer is not clear. First, one cannot ignore psychologic function and focus only on musculoskeletal function. Second, the functional value of a limb following resection must be compared with the functional value of the available alternatives. Most surgeons recognize that a below-the-knee amputation offers such good function that patients with tumors distal to the midtibia are best treated by amputation. Upper extremity prostheses provide little compared to the normal hand, so patients with lesions of the proximal humerus are undoubtedly best treated by resection, regardless of age. The development of total hip replacement arthroplasty has evolved to such an extent that patients with tumors of the proximal one-third of the femur will often be treated best by resection.

It is in lesions of the distal femur and proximal tibia that the choice of resection vs amputation is most difficult. Children under the age of 12 or 13 are not usually appropriate candidates for resection of distal femoral lesions because of the marked leg-length discrepancy which will result. The massive skin flaps following resection require careful nurturing. Concern for skin healing may delay postoperative exercises sufficiently that ultimate knee flexion may be very limited. Of the twelve patients with resections in the knee area in our series, six have 70 to 90 degrees of knee flexion, three have approximately 30 degrees, and three have less than 30 degrees. That this is sufficient for a vigorous teenager is doubtful; yet few orthopedic surgeons would treat limited knee-motion secondary to nonneoplastic disease by amputation. It will take a number of years for adequate follow-up studies to determine the appropriate surgical treatment for these lesions.

Arthrodesis as described by Enneking is a useful alternative; however, most children prefer some knee motion to none.[8] We have used arthrodesis in four patients with proximal tibial lesions but have used an intramedullary rod with methylmethacrylate cement and stainless steel mesh to obviate the problems of bone healing secondary to high-dose methotrexate. We now prefer this option in proximal tibital lesions, where there is so little soft tissue to cover an articulated metal endoprosthesis.

EWING'S SARCOMA

For a number of years, radiation has been the usual first choice for treatment of the primary lesion in Ewing's sarcoma. Ewing's sarcomas in the foot, however, have customarily been treated by surgery, since the tissues of the sole of the foot respond poorly to radiation therapy.

Recently there has been a growing concern that radiation is not adequate and that primary Ewing's tumors in the lower extremity should be treated by amputation. There are several reasons for this. One is that radiation often leaves a functionally limited extremity. There is also concern about late recurrence of tumor (for up to 12 years following radiation) and postirradiation sarcoma.

Radiation, at doses sufficient for treating Ewing's sarcoma, is virtually certain to cause growth arrest of the femur or tibia if the epiphyses are included in the field. In younger children who survive, the marked limb-length inequality may require a subsequent amputation. However, the long-term survival of Ewing's tumor patients treated with radiation therapy and adjuvant chemotherapy is still in question, and it is probably more humane to postpone amputation until survival for five years has been attained. Prior to that time, the limb inequality can readily be handled by appropriate shoe lifts.

Proponents of surgical ablation of lower extremity Ewing's sarcoma agree that upper extremity lesions should still be treated by radiation because of the better function of an intact hand compared to a prosthesis.

If a fracture occurs through an irradiated bone and the patient is receiving chemotherapy, healing of the fracture cannot be expected until the chemotherapy course—frequently two or more years—is completed. Such fractures require internal fixation. Treatment by traction will impede radiation treatment as well as lead to further osteoporosis, complicating the ultimate internal fixation. Excessive bleeding has not been a feature of these operations and should not deter the surgeon from using internal fixation. Occasionally, amputation for pathologic fracture of a weight-bearing bone may have to be considered.

REFERENCES

1. Dahlin, D. and Coventry, M.: Osteogenic sarcoma: a study of 600 cases. *J Bone Joint Surg* 49A:101, 1967.

2. Jaffe, N.: The potential for combined modality approaches. *Cancer Treat Rev* 2:33–53, 1975.

3. Sweetnam, R.: Osteosarcoma. *Ann R Coll Surg* 44:38, 1968.

4. Coventry, M. and Dahlin, D.: Osteogenic sarcoma: a critical analysis of 430 cases. *J Bone Joint Surg* 39A:741, 1957.

5. Lee, E.S. and MacKenzie, D.: Osteosarcoma: a study of the value of preoperative megavoltage radiotherapy. *Br J Surg* 51:252, 1964.

6. Moore, G., Gertner, R., and Brugarolus, A.: Osteogenic sarcoma. *Surg Gynecol Obstet* 136:359, 1973.

7. Enneking, W.F. and Kagan, A.: 'Skip' metastases in osteosarcoma. *Cancer* 36:2192, 1975.

8. Enneking, W.F. and Shirley, P.D.: Resection-arthrodesis for malignant and potentially malignant lesions about the knee using intramedullary rod and local bone grafts. *J Bone Joint Surg* 49A:223, 1977.

9 En Bloc Resection and Prosthetic Replacement in Osteosarcoma

Ralph C. Marcove, M.D.

Preservation of a limb without sacrificing the principles of cancer surgery is a desirable goal in a young patient with osteosarcoma. At the present time, amputation is regarded by most authorities as the only well-established curative treatment for this malignancy.[1-6] For a tumor close to a joint, amputation usually includes excision of a part of the adjacent joint bone as well as much of the involved bone to ensure that both potential capsular local spread and possible intraosseous skip areas of tumor are removed. The distal femur lesion, which has the lowest cure rate usually involves removing the whole bone.[7]

The following study was undertaken to determine whether en bloc resection in association with intensive chemotherapy is a realistic alternative to radical amputation and chemotherapy.[8-14] This chapter presents a preliminary report on 43 patients who underwent en bloc resection for osteosarcoma of the femur (20 patients), tibia (11 patients), shoulder girdle (11 patients), and fibula (1 patient).

MATERIALS AND METHODS

All patients underwent routine history-taking, physical examinations, and laboratory determinations. Standard AP and lateral x-rays of the involved bone, as well as skeletal survey, bone scan, and chest tomography, were performed. Biplane arteriography of the osteosarcomatous area was done (Figure 1).[15] [16] All data were evaluated to determine the size, location, and resectability of the tumor and its soft tissue components, as well as the presence or absence of metastatic disease or skip areas. In children with distal femur lesions, orthoroentgenographic scanograms of the lower extremities, and appropriate studies to determine the degree of skeletal maturity and projected growth curves, were also done. The objectives and potential risks of the treatment protocol were carefully explained to the participants and their families. The presence of pulmonary metastases was not necessarily a contraindication as long as the lesions appeared surgically resectable and/or responsive to chemotherapy.[14] [17-22] The advisability of using an ischial weight-bearing brace postoperatively was discussed with the parents and patients before surgery.

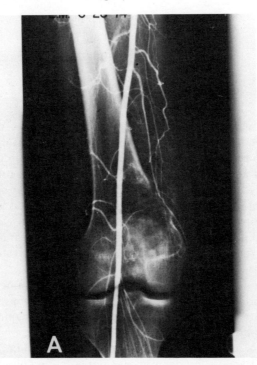

Figure 1A. Arteriograph of distal femoral osteosarcoma, showing resectability of lesion.

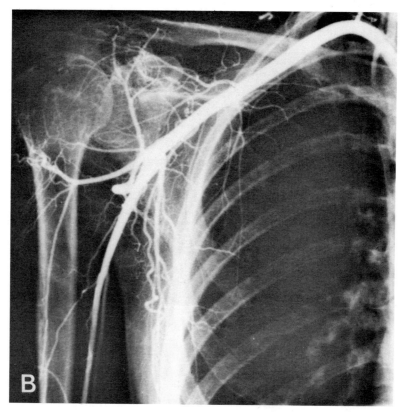

Figure 1B. Arteriograph of osteosarcomatous scapula lesion, showing resectability of lesion.

DISTAL FEMUR LESIONS

Once the initial work-up—including scanograms, routine physical examinations, and x-ray examinations—is complete, construction of the metal total femur with a total knee prosthesis begins. This construction takes approximately eight weeks. During this time the patient is maintained on a chemotherapeutic regimen consisting of vincristine, Adriamycin, and high-dose methotrexate with citrovorum "rescue."[14] [21] [22] When the prosthesis is ready the patient is reevaluated: if the protocol criteria are still valid, the replacement is performed. After sufficient postoperative wound healing, adjuvant chemotherapy resumes, consisting of biweekly cyclophosphamide, vincristine, high-dose methotrexate and citrovorum rescue, and Adriamycin for five cycles. Immediately after surgery, the patient is placed in a long-leg ischial weight-bearing brace (at first with a pelvic band) and started on active range-of-motion exercises, as well as ambulation, as the clinical situation allows. The pelvic band portion is removed in about six weeks (Figure 2).

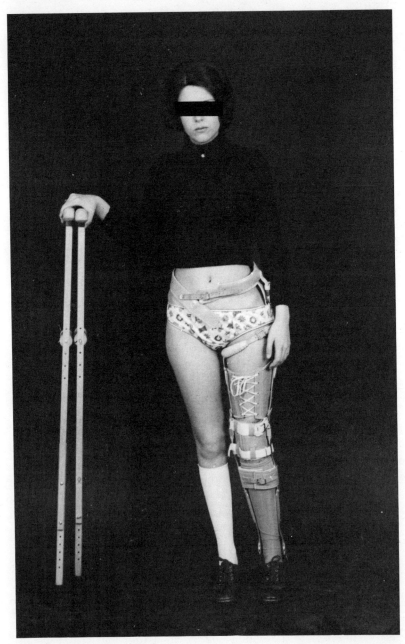

Figure 2. Patient in ischial weight-bearing brace with pelvic band after total femur and knee replacement.

Operative Technique

A lateral biopsy approach is used in previously untreated cases where this is the proposed site of the subsequent surgical incision. Through a long Gibson skin incision, posterior and anterior approaches are made into the hip on the affected side. The incision itself is carried along the greater trochanter down the lateral aspect of the femur distal to the knee. The incision is then curved slightly anteriorly over the proximal lateral tibia to extend 4 cm distal to the tibial tubercle. The previous biopsy scar and tract are included in the surgical resection. The incision is carried through the layers, and as the resection nears the area of tumor, ample margin is left on the femur so that tumor is never seen. If tumor pseudocapsule is encountered during surgery, the operation is discontinued and, after a change of instruments, a higher level of amputation is performed. (This occurred once in the study under discussion.)

The knee is removed en bloc with the distal femur. The patella tendon is maintained intact and the patella is split coronally so that the inner half stays with the specimen and the outer half remains in continuity with the retained quadriceps mechanism. The tibia is reamed to accept the stem of the total knee prosthesis, and methyl methacrylate is placed in the tibia after a trial reduction of the prosthesis (Figure 3). The glutei are attached with heavy silk through preformed holes in the prosthetic shaft proximally, and the medial and lateral thigh muscles are attached to each other. The distal hamstrings are often transferred anteriorly to act as knee extensors and to help give a deep layer below the skin incision. The wound is carefully checked for hemostasis (cautery is usually not used), and closure with hemovacs is accomplished. The patient is placed on prophylactic antibiotics preoperatively and postoperatively, and the wound is flushed with local antibiotics during and immediately after surgery. The leg is elevated postoperatively.

Results

Twenty-six patients with distal femur lesions were originally considered for replacement surgery.[23] Of these, 5 were started on the protocol described, but because of the tumor size, amputations were performed. One patient was amputated at the time of surgery, as tumor pseudocapsule was encountered.

As shown in Figure 4, the 20 remaining patients, ages 11 to 21, have been followed up for 2 to 35 months. Thirteen patients (65%) are alive and disease-free; one patient is alive with disease. Nine (52%) of 17 patients admitted to protocol disease-free are still without disease.

148

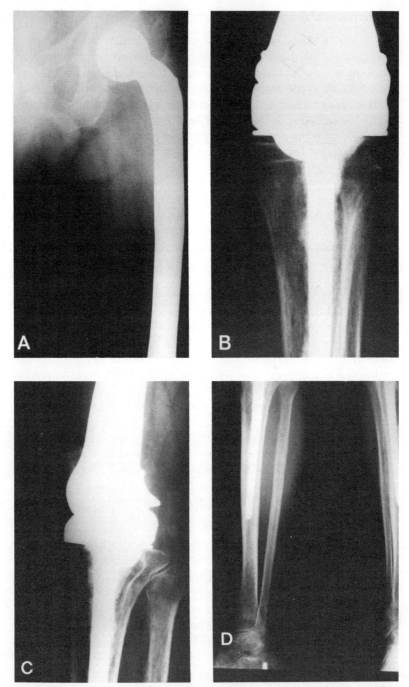

Figure 3. Postoperative x-rays showing total femur (**A**) and knee (**B, C,** and **D**) replacements in place.

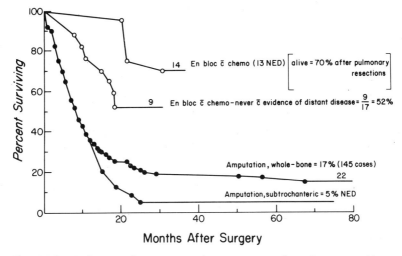

Figure 4. Survival curves of 20 patients with osteosarcoma who underwent total femur resections with chemotherapy (with and without pulmonary surgery); 17 patients were admitted with only localized disease. The results of amputation and en bloc femur resection are compared. Adapted from Marcove et al.[7]

Of the three patients admitted with pulmonary lesions, one is alive now without disease at 24 months postreplacement (she had a second pulmonary metastasis and thoracotomy at 7 months postreplacement); the other two patients expired at 21 and 30 months, respectively, with widespread metastases. Six patients underwent thoracotomies; 3 are alive without disease. One patient had a negative exploratory thoracotomy after chemotherapy had shrunk her nodule.

Seven patients needed amputations: three for infection, two for local recurrence, one for prosthesis breakage, and one for radiation necrosis (6,600 rad had been given prior to replacement). Of the three in this group who are now alive and disease-free, one had infection; one had a local recurrence; and one experienced mechanical failure.

Functional Results

Walking progressed from the use of crutches to the assistance of a cane. Without a cane, a gluteus maximus limp is observed unless an ischial weight-bearing brace is used. Ranges of motion usually improve with time; ankle and foot motion usually is quite good. Patients are instructed to wear the ischial weight-bearing brace with quadrilateral socket and to treat the extremity much the same as a "polio leg."

SHOULDER GIRDLE LESIONS

The Tikhoff-Linberg procedure (en bloc upper humeral, interscapulothoracic resection) is an alternative to radical ablation for neoplasms of the shoulder girdle.[24-30] Resection may be attempted if the neoplasm does not involve the axillary artery or the brachial plexus; if lymph nodes are negative; and if the neoplasm is not fixed in the chest wall. Primary tumors of bone, as well as soft tissue tumors adjacent to the bone, can be treated by this method. However, a forequarter amputation is probably a better operation if lymph nodes are involved.[5 30]

Operative Technique

The initial incision is made along the inner two-thirds of the clavicle and is then extended distally from the region of the coracoid along the medial border of the arm over the neurovascular bundle. Posteriorly, one extends the incision longitudinally in the midscapular region. The incision is altered so that the biopsy scar and tract is excised with the specimen. If the neurovascular bundle is free of tumor, the mobilization of the neurovascular bundle continues. The musculocutaneous and radial nerves can be identified and are usually preserved. If, however, the lesion involves the soft tissue of the nerve in the vicinity of the proximal humerus, the radial and the musculocutaneous nerves may have to be sacrificed. In one case, even the ulnar nerve was removed, leaving the hand with only a median nerve.

The posterior skin incision originates at the lateral third of the clavicle and is carried posteriorly and longitudinally along the midscapula to the angle of the scapula. The inferior angle of the scapula is mobilized and the entire vertebral border is resected from the chest wall, similarly to the plane developed in the forequarter amputation. For lesions of the scapula, a wide soft tissue margin must be maintained. The skin flap from the initial incision is raised over the proximal humerus; the deltoid is left intact with the specimen in upper humeral lesions.

When much of the humerus is removed, excessive shortening can be avoided and better elbow power for flexion can be provided by fixating a humeral prosthesis or Küntscher nail replacement into the proximal soft tissue or the clavicle stump (Figure 5). Some patients are more comfortable if a greater amount of clavicle is removed and nail fixation is into the soft tissue. Hemovacs are placed in the wound and closure is routine. A postoperative sling and a swathe or Valpeau dressing are employed. Hand and elbow range of motion exercises are encouraged soon after the operation.

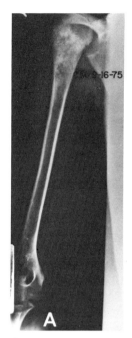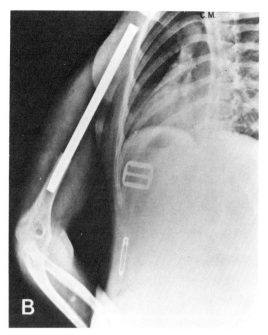

Figure 5. (A) Preoperative radiograph of osteosarcoma of the humerus in an 11-year-old girl. **(B)** Postoperative film showing Küntscher nail inserted after resection to maintain length of arm in same patient.

Results

Thirty-seven Tikhoff-Linberg procedures have been performed. Eleven of these cases were done for osteosarcoma.[31] The patients ranged in age from 8 to 63 and their tumor was in the shoulder girdle (upper end of the humerus, scapula, and clavicle). Follow-up is from 2 to 37 months. Seven patients (63%) are alive without evidence of disease (Figure 6). One patient of this group was admitted with pulmonary metastases, and thoracotomies were performed at 2, 7, and 13 months postresection. He is now (3 months after the last thoracotomy) without evidence of disease.

Of the four patients who died, one had been admitted with pulmonary metastases (radiation osteosarcoma from previous Hodgkin's disease) and died of widespread metastatic disease 6 months postresection. Surgery in this case was for palliative purposes only. Another patient died 7 months postresection with widespread disease and a local recurrence. The local recurrence could not have been improved by a forequarter amputation because the same tissue planes—those at the levator scapula—would have given trouble. The other two patients died of widespread metastases.

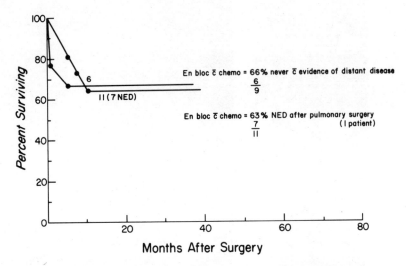

Figure 6. Survival curves for 11 patients who underwent Tikhoff-Linberg procedures and chemotherapy (with and without pulmonary surgery) for osteosarcomas of the shoulder girdle.

Six patients (66%) never had any evidence of distant disease. One patient in this group was given postoperative vaccine (lysed cell) therapy four years ago. Only five patients in this group were included in the chemotherapy program and all are free of disease, including the one patient who had three thoracotomies.

Functional Results

Wrist and hand function is normal in this group. In those with radial nerve palsy, a cock-up splint was used and tendon transfers were done two years after the initial surgery. A small amount of shoulder padding usually corrects the surgical deformity under clothing, but a plastic filler is ideal for this purpose.

PROXIMAL TIBIA LESIONS

As in patients with lesions of the shoulder girdle or distal femur, appropriate preoperative work-up is done to determine resectability of proximal tibia lesions. Again, this includes bone age studies, chest tomography, and biplane arteriography. Skeletal survey and bone scans are done to rule out any distant lesions. After the en bloc resection and total long-stem knee replacement, patients are started on the chemotherapy protocol.[9] [14] [21]

Operative Technique

A posterior medial incision is made and the neurovascular bundle is identified. The anterior tibial artery, as well as other interosseous, perforating vessels, are ligated at the posterior tibial vessel. The popliteal fossa vessels are also ligated, preserving the main stem. The fibula is removed en bloc, along with the upper tibia (for tumor in the latter, because of its proximity). For total knee replacement, the distal femur is also removed en bloc, keeping a margin of normal tissue planes around the tumor. Care must be taken to preserve cutaneous nerves. If the upper tibia in the subcutaneous region has tumor growing into the skin, this area, of course, must be sacrificed. The long-stem Guepar knee (with solid shafts) is cemented into the residual distal tibia and proximal femur.

Results

Eleven patients, aged 11 to 24 years, with lesions of the proximal tibia and a follow-up of 4 to 23 months, were included in this group (Figure 7). Eight patients (72%) have never had any evidence of distant disease. Two patients are alive with disease after having had thoracotomies at 16 and 20 months postresection, respectively. One patient died 3 months after surgery with pulmonary metastases and local recurrence. In retrospect, her lesion was too large to have been operable. One patient was amputated, at his request, because of excessive numbness of his foot (too many cutaneous nerves had been sacrificed).

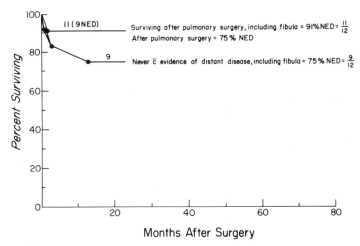

Figure 7. Survival curves of 12 patients, 11 with tibia lesions and one with fibula lesion, treated with en bloc resection of tibia and fibula together with chemotherapy, with and without pulmonary surgery.

FIBULA LESION

A 15-year-old female who had sustained a direct blow below the right knee three weeks prior to admission, and who experienced continued mild discomfort and swelling, was referred to our institution. Radiographs revealed an osteosarcoma of the right fibula. The right knee joint had a full range of motion. Clinically, the lateral popliteal nerve was intact. Further routine work-up was normal, and an arteriogram showed resectability of "tumor." She was started on a chemotherapeutic regimen, and surgery was performed after a frozen-section biopsy had been done.

Operative Technique

A long skin incision was made from above the knee joint to the ankle, leaving a segment of skin directly overlying the tumor. Skin flaps were developed anteriorly and posteriorly. Dissection was deepened. The tumor was never encountered, and a 2-cm normal margin was left over the tumor. (Consent had been obtained for a midthigh amputation if the tumor pseudocapsule were seen.) The lower fibula was disarticulated at the ankle mortice. With the use of an osteotome, a rim of tibia above and medial to the tibiofibular joint, including part of the lateral tibial condyle, was removed en bloc with the specimen. Thus, the whole of the fibula, the tumor, the tibiofibular joint, a wide surrounding margin of muscles, and the common peroneal nerve were removed en bloc. Two of the three lower limb arteries were ligated. A long-leg plaster of paris cast was applied, with the ankle in the neutral position, for six weeks. Later, stress views showed no instability.

Results

Because of persistent fluid collection, chemotherapy was delayed for two months after surgery. Vincristine, methotrexate, and citrovorum "rescue" were given according to our adjuvant chemotherapy protocol, and this treatment was continued for one year.[14][21][22] The patient walked without a limp with a drop foot brace and was free of disease for two and a half years. A nodule then developed inside the upper tibia, and the remaining upper tibia was therefore removed en bloc. A Guepar total knee with long-stem prosthesis was inserted. The patient is well postoperatively, and there is good stability of the ankle joint. The residual capsule, as well as the lateral ligaments, contribute to the lateral stability of the ankle joint.

SUMMARY AND CONCLUSIONS

In all, 43 patients have been treated for osteosarcoma of the extremities by en bloc resection and chemotherapy; some have also undergone pulmonary resections. Seventy-four percent of this group are alive after tumor resection, chemotherapy, and pulmonary resections; to date, 67% are alive with no evidence of disease after the above treatment (Figure 8).

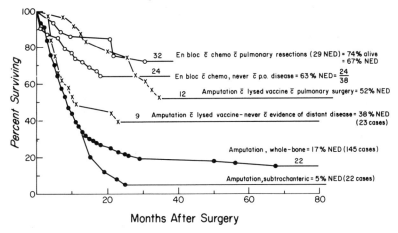

Figure 8. Survival curves of 43 patients with osteosarcoma, comparing results of amputation to treatment with en bloc resections and chemotherapy (with and without pulmonary surgery). Adapted from Marcove et al.[7]

Twenty-four (63%) of 38 patients (5 of the 43 are excluded from consideration here because they initially presented with pulmonary lesions) are alive without evidence of disease and have never manifested distant disease postoperatively. Comparison of published survival curves show these results considerably better than those obtained with previously described treatment plans. Previous studies report 52% NED (no evidence of disease) after amputation, lysed cell vaccine, and pulmonary surgery; 38% NED after amputation and lysed cell vaccine in those who had never shown evidence of distant disease; 17% NED after whole-bone amputation; and 5% NED after subtrochanteric amputation. (Figure 8).[7]

The ultimate test for this surgery is the control of tumor. The previously reported mean time for development of pulmonary metastases after amputation for osteosarcoma was 7.9 months.[32] In a recent study at the Memorial Sloan-Kettering Cancer Center, x-rays were taken more frequently postoperatively—at one-month intervals—and the mean time for detecting pulmonary metastases was 5.5 months.[20] Poor survival statistics in spite of adequate radical ablation of the primary tumor site in childhood osteosarcoma are probably due to the presence of distant microfoci of disease, usually pulmonary, at the time of surgery.[33] [34] Hence, there is need for pulmonary resections and for systemic chemotherapy with drugs with demonstrated efficacy against this radioresistant tumor.

Limb preservation is being investigated by use of cryosurgery and/or en bloc excision. Cryosurgery may be tried for giant cell tumors and low-grade chondrosarcomas. Ewing's sarcoma is also being treated with chemotherapy, en bloc resection, and low-dose radiotherapy, preoperatively or postoperatively. This is done to avoid the damaging effects and high morbidity rate that accompany treatment by high doses of radiation alone, as well as to reduce the significant number of local tumor recurrences observed with standard treatment.

Even though our results with en bloc replacement surgery have been favorable so far, long-term survival data are still not available. Therefore, it is advisable to undertake this procedure only in a major institution where facilities are available for proper evaluation and follow-up. This therapy should, of course, be coordinated with other types of treatment that may be necessary.

REFERENCES

1. Dahlin, D.C. and Coventry, M.B.: Osteosarcoma: a study of 600 cases. *J Bone Joint Surg* 49A:101, 1967.

2. Francis, K.C., Hutter, R.V.P., and Coley, B.C.: Treatment of osteogenic sarcoma. In Pack, G. and Ariel, J. (eds): *Treatment of Cancer and Allied Diseases,* Vol. 8. Harper & Row, New York, 1964, pp 374–399.

3. Lewis, R.J. and Lotz, M.J.: Medullary extension of osteosarcoma. *Cancer* 33:371, 1974.

4. Miller, T.R.: Eleven cases of hemipelvectomy: a personal experience. *Surg Clin North Am* 54:913, 1974.

5. Pack, G.T., McNeer, G., and Coley, B.L.: Interscapulothoracic amputation for malignant tumors of the upper extremity: a report of 31 consecutive cases. *Surg Gynecol Obstet* 74:161, 1942.

6. Sweetnam, R.: Amputation in osteosarcoma. *J Bone Joint Surg* 55B:189, 1973.

7. Marcove, R.C., Mike, V., Hajek, J.V. et al: Osteogenic sarcoma in childhood. *NY State J Med* 71:855, 1971.

8. Bingold, A.C.: Prosthetic replacement of a chondrosarcoma of the upper end of the femur: 18-year follow-up. *J Bone Joint Surg* 54B:139, 1972.

9. Huvos, A.G., Rosen, G., and Marcove, R.C.: Pathologic aspects of primary osteogenic sarcoma treated by chemotherapy, en

bloc resection, and prosthetic bone replacement: a study of twenty patients. *Arch Pathol Lab Med* 101:14, 1977.

10. Marcove, R.C.: New trends in the treatment of osteogenic sarcoma. *Orthop Digest* 3:11, 1975.

11. Marcove, R.C. and Khafagy, M.M.: Total femur and knee replacement using a metallic prosthesis. *Clin Bull* 4:69, 1974.

12. Ottolenghi, C.E.: Massive osteoarticular bone grafts: transplant of the whole femur. *J Bone Joint Surg* 48B:646, 1966.

13. Parrish, F.F.: Allograft replacement of all or part of the end of a long bone following excision of a tumor: report of 21 cases. *J Bone Joint Surg* 55A: 1, 1973.

14. Rosen, G., Murphy, M.L., Huvos, A.G. et al: Chemotherapy, en bloc resection, and prosthetic bone replacement in the treatment of osteogenic sarcoma. *Cancer* 37:1, 1976.

15. Hollinshead, W.H.: *Anatomy for Surgeons Volume 3: Back and Limbs.* 2d ed. Harper & Row Publishers, Inc., New York, 1969, p 830.

16. Hudson, T., Hass, G., Enneking, W. et al: Angiography in the management of musculoskeletal tumors. *Surg Gynecol Obstet* 141:11, 1975.

17. Beattie, E.J., Jr., Rosen, G., and Martini, N.: The management of pulmonary metastases in children with osteogenic sarcoma with surgical resection combined with chemotherapy. *Cancer* 35:618, 1975.

18. Marcove, R.C. and Lewis, M.M.: Prolonged survival in osteogenic sarcoma with pulmonary metastases. *J Bone Joint Surg* 55A:1516, 1973.

19. Marcove, R.C., Martini, N., and Rosen, G.: The treatment of pulmonary metastasis in osteogenic sarcoma. *Clin Orthop* 111:65, 1975.

20. Martini, N., Huvos, A.G., Mike, V. et al: Multiple pulmonary resections in the treatment of osteogenic sarcoma. *Ann Thorac Surg* 12:271, 1971.

21. Rosen, G., Suwansirikul, S., Kwon, C. et al: High-dose methotrexate with citrovorum factor rescue and Adriamycin in childhood osteogenic sarcoma. *Cancer* 33:115, 1974.

22. Rosen, G., Tan, C., Sanmaneechai, A. et al: The rationale for multiple drug chemotherapy in the treatment of osteogenic sarcoma. *Cancer* 35:936, 1975.

23. Marcove, R.C., Lewis, M.M., Rosen, G. et al: Total femur replacement. *Compr Ther* 3:13, 1977.

24. Burnel, H.N.: Resection of the shoulder with humeral suspension for sarcoma involving the scapula. *J Bone Joint Surg.* 47B:300, 1965.

25. Francis, K.C. and Worcester, J.N.: Radical resection for tumors of the shoulder with preservation of a functional extremity. *J Bone Joint Surg* 44A:1423, 1962.

26. Linberg, B.E.: Interscapulothoracic resection for malignant tumors of the shoulder joint region. *J Bone Joint Surg* 10:344, 1928.

27. Janeck, C.J. and Nelson, C.L.: En bloc resection of the shoulder girdle: technique and indications. Report of a case. *J Bone Joint Surg* 54A:1754, 1972.

28. Marcove, R.C.: Neoplasms of the shoulder girdle. *Orthop Clin North Am* 6:541, 1975.

29. Pack, G.T. and Baldwin, J.C.: The Tikhoff-Linberg resection of shoulder girdle: case report. *Surgery* 38:753, 1955.

30. Samilson, R.L., Morris, J.M., and Thompson, R.W.: Tumors of the scapula. *Clin Orthop* 58:105, 1968.

31. Marcove, R.C., Lewis, M.M., and Huvos, A.G.: En bloc upper humeral interscapulothoracic resection: the Tikhoff-Linberg procedure. *Clin Orthop* 124:219, 1977.

32. Marcove, R.C., Mike, V., Hajek, J.V. et al: Osteogenic sarcoma under the age of 21: a review of 145 operative cases. *J Bone Joint Surg* 52A:411, 1970.

33. Jaffe, N., Farber, S., Traggis, D. et al: Favorable response of metastatic osteogenic sarcoma to pulse high-dose methotrexate with citrovorum rescue and radiation therapy. *Cancer* 31:1367, 1973.

34. Ohno, T., Mitsutoshi, A., Tateishi, A. et al: Osteogenic sarcoma: a study of 130 cases. *J Bone Joint Surg* 57A:397, 1975.

10 En Bloc Resection and Allograft Replacement for Osteosarcoma of the Extremity

Frederick R. Eilber, M.D.
Donald L. Morton, M.D.
Todd T. Grant, M.D.

1. Clinical and treatment data
   a. Preoperative treatment
   b. Surgical procedure
   c. Adjuvant chemotherapy
2. Results and complications
3. Histologic evaluation
4. Discussion

The standard surgical therapy for osteosarcoma of bone has been amputation. The only controversy over the surgical management has concerned the level at which to amputate. Most surgeons would recommend amputation of the extremity one joint above the site of the primary tumor to prevent local recurrence, although in one large series, amputation through the shaft of the bone has been accomplished with comparable results.[1] There have been few previous attempts to perform en bloc resection of the involved bone with allograft replacement, and they have usually resulted in failure.* However, review of these cases shows that the majority of the treatment failures were due not to recurrent tumors at the primary site but to distant, pulmonary metastases. In an effort to avoid amputation, Cade attempted high-dose radiation therapy to the primary tumor in the small percentage of patients who did not develop metastases.[2] Although this therapy did not improve the overall survival rates, amputation could be avoided in approximately 90% of these patients and there were a few long-term survivors.

*Investigations reported in this chapter were supported by grant CA-12582 and contract CB-53941, awarded by the National Cancer Institute, (DHEW) and by the Medical Research Service of the Veterans Administration.

The results of clinical trials of chemotherapy for osteosarcoma have demonstrated its effectiveness. Significant therapeutic benefit against established metastatic disease has been derived from Adriamycin and high-dose methotrexate. These drugs have significantly reduced the incidence of distant disease when used as adjuvants in postamputation treatment regimens.[3-7] Rosen et al have reconsidered the problem of the primary tumor in light of this evidence.[8] They have employed these chemotherapeutic agents before the operation and report an 80% success rate for radical en bloc excision of the primary tumor. The involved bone was replaced with a metallic endoprosthesis.

Encouraged by these results, we began a clinical trial in an effort to incorporate all the known modalities for treatment of this tumor. We began in 1976 with preoperative intra-arterial Adriamycin chemotherapy and rapid-fraction radiation, followed by en bloc excision of the involved bone and surrounding soft tissue. Bone replacement was achieved with a cadaver allograft.

CLINICAL AND TREATMENT DATA

Twenty-four patients with osteosarcoma of the extremity (all biopsy-proven) were evaluated by the Divisions of Surgical Oncology and Orthopedics of the University of California at Los Angeles School of Medicine from September 1974 to September 1977. All patients were advised that the standard method of therapy was amputation but that, if they refused, an experimental protocol for attempted limb preservation was available. Sixteen of the 24 patients refused amputation. This group was treated with preoperative intra-arterial Adriamycin and radiation therapy, followed by radical en bloc excision of their primary tumor and cadaver allograft. Eight patients elected the standard operation, which involves amputation of the extremity one joint above the site of the primary tumor.

Of the 16 patients who elected limb preservation, there were 10 males and 6 females, ranging in age from 12 to 49 years (median: 17 years). The sites of their primary tumors comprised: femur, 10; ilium, 2; and humerus, 4 (Table 1). There were 4 males and 4 females treated by amputation, and they ranged in age from 3 to 32 years (median: 17 years). Their primary tumors were located in: femur, 4; ilium, 2; tibia, 1; and humerus, 1.

Preoperative Treatment

Those patients who refused amputation underwent percu-

Table 1
Osteosarcoma: Clinical Characteristics of Treatment Groups

No. of Patients	Limb Preservation Group	Amputation Group
Age range (years)	16	8
Sex	12-49 (17)*	3-32 (17)*
Male	10	4
Female	6	4
Tumor location		
Femur	10	4
Ilium	2	2
Tibia	0	1
Humerus	4	1

*Number in parentheses represents median age.

taneous arteriography to ascertain the vasculature and extramedullary extent of the tumor. A Silastic catheter was inserted for drug infusion. A 30-mg dose of Adriamycin in 50 cc of saline solution was infused (by a Harvard pump) over a 24-hour period for three consecutive days, for a total dose of 90 mg. Immediately after infusion, radiation therapy was begun. A 6-meV linear accelerator delivered 350 rad/day for 10 days, for a total dose of 3,500 rad to the midplane in ten equal fractions over 12 to 15 calendar days. This radiation dose, delivered by rapid fractionation, is comparable to 4,800 rad given by standard dose fractions. The portals were posteroanterior and anteroposterior, parallel, opposed fields, and both fields were treated daily. The portals included the entire region of the tumor. A strip of skin opposite the primary tumor was spared.

Surgical Procedure

Surgical resection was performed one week after completion of the radiotherapy. Ten femurs and four humeri were replaced with cadaver allografts obtained from the tissue bank of the National Naval Medical Center, Bethesda, Maryland. These allografts had been removed under sterile conditions, irradiated, and preserved by freeze-drying. Preoperatively, attempts were made to match intracondylar and intramedullary diameters of the recipient bones with the allografts by comparison to nonmagnified radiographs.

Radical en bloc excision of the bone and surrounding musculature was performed. Major blood vessels and nerves were dissected on a subadventitial plane and preserved. A proximal margin of 10 cm was achieved in all resections, and the proximal bone marrow was curetted and examined by frozen section for evidence of tumor. The femoral allografts were internally fixed with a Sampson intramedullary rod. Collateral ligaments at the knee joints and elbows were reattached with staples and no attempt was made to achieve cruciate or capsular repairs. Patients with femoral allografts were placed in long-leg casts and were ambulated non-weight-bearing for eight weeks. An ischial weight-bearing long-leg brace then replaced the cast.

Adjuvant Chemotherapy

All 24 patients with osteosarcoma were treated postoperatively with Adriamycin and high-dose methotrexate. The adjuvant chemotherapy was begun one week after the surgical procedure. Vincristine was given intravenously at a dose of 1.5 mg/M^2 one hour before a 4-hour infusion of methotrexate (initial dose: 100 mg/kg). Four hours following completion of the methotrexate infusion, citrovorum rescue was started, at a dosage of 12 mg every 6 hours for three days. Methotrexate serum levels were measured at 24 and 48 hours postinfusion.[9] Two weeks after methotrexate administration, 45 mg/M^2 of Adriamycin was given as an intravenous bolus on each of two consecutive days, for a total treatment dose of 90 mg/M^2. Two weeks after the Adriamycin treatment, 200 mg/kg of methotrexate was given, and the cycle (methotrexate-Adriamycin) was repeated until a cumulative dose of 500 mg/M^2 of Adriamycin was achieved. Adriamycin then was discontinued and high-dose methotrexate was given once monthly for an additional six months, to a total adjuvant treatment time of one year.

RESULTS AND COMPLICATIONS

The overall results of treatment for the 24 patients are shown in Table 2. Of the 8 patients treated by amputation and adjuvant chemotherapy, 5 (62%) are free of disease and 3 had recurrence of their disease. One patient had successful treatment of pulmonary metastases, and two patients expired: one from local recurrence (primary site: ilium) and one from distant disease. The median follow-up time for patients in the amputation group was 12.0 months.

Of the 16 patients treated by intra-arterial Adriamycin-radiation therapy and allograft replacement, 11 (69%) are free of disease. Five patients experienced recurrent disease. One of the 5 had local recurrence which was successfully treated by amputation; the remaining 4 developed pulmonary metastases (which were surgically resected), and one expired from recurrent disease in the chest. Follow-up time in this group was 3 to 26 months (median: 13.5 months).

Table 2
Osteosarcoma: Overall Treatment Results

	Treatment of Primary Tumor		
	Intra-arterial Adriamycin + Radiotherapy and Allograft	Amputation	Total
No. of patients	16	8	24
No evidence of disease at follow-up*	11 (69)	5 (62)	16 (67)
With recurrence at follow-up†	5	3	8
Expired	1	2	3

*3 to 26 months posttreatment (median: 13.5 months.) Numbers in parentheses represent percentages.
†2 to 36 months posttreatment (median: 12.0 months).

Functional knee motion is minimal in the 10 patients who received femoral allografts. Surprisingly, these patients have medial and lateral stability but no anteroposterior stability. However, stability in the anteroposterior plane has been achieved with a pretibial shell on the long-leg orthosis. The average arc of flexion for these patients is 10 to 15 degrees, and all have full extension power. The 4 patients who had upper extremity allografts have progressed the most satisfactorily. Elbow motion of as much as 34 degrees has been achieved. Hand and wrist motion is normal, but one patient has only negligible shoulder mobility.

Three (18%) of the 16 patients treated by preoperative Adriamycin-radiation therapy developed major complications. One patient who has had a deep infection at the site of the allograft, and intermittently draining sinuses which have required antibiotics and packing over 21 months refuses amputation and continues to ambulate on the extremity. Another patient developed a local recurrence near the resection site that required amputation. This is the only incidence of local tumor recurrence that we have encountered. Upon review of the specimens from this case, it was apparent that the primary femoral tumor involved the joint capsule and that the disease probably spread by direct extension to the tibia. The third patient with complications required amputation at 9 months postresection because of a femoral artery thrombosis secondary to proliferative intimitis. A femoral artery graft was attempted but was unsuccessful.

HISTOLOGIC EVALUATION

To evaluate the effect of preoperative Adriamycin and radiation therapy on tumor histology, pretreatment biopsy and posttreatment tumor specimens were compared. Tumor cell necrosis was estimated visually on 10 to 12 slides per specimen and was defined as total absence of identifiable nuclei. Evaluation of the postoperative specimen was made without knowledge of the type of preoperative therapy given. The degree of tumor cell necrosis was then correlated with the type of preoperative therapy administered.

The benefits of preoperative intra-arterial Adriamycin and radiation therapy were confirmed by histologic examination. Specimens from those patients who had been amputated showed an average tumor cell necrosis of 15%. Although there was some variation in the range of the natural incidence of tumor cell necrosis, spontaneous necrosis rarely exceeded 30%. Preoperative Adriamycin infusion and radiation therapy, however yielded dramatic histologic evidence, with an average tumor cell necrosis of 86%, and no viable tumor cells were seen in four specimens (Table 3).

Table 3
Influence of Preoperative Chemotherapy and Radiation Therapy on the Incidence of Necrosis in Osteosarcoma Specimens

| | Incidence of Necrosis (%) | | |
Treatment	Patients	Range	Average
Amputation followed by chemotherapy	8	0–30	15
Preoperative Adriamycin and radiation therapy with en bloc resection and allograft replacement	16	80–100*	86

*Four specimens showed no viable tumor cells.

DISCUSSION

The impact of an effective chemotherapeutic regimen on the clinical course of patients with malignant osteosarcoma is evident. Long-term follow-up of the patients who were initially treated by adjuvant chemotherapy indicates that approximately 50% to 60% will remain free of recurrent disease for at least nine months (Figure 1).

CUMULATIVE PERCENT OF PATIENTS WITH OSTEOSARCOMA FREE OF RECURRENT DISEASE

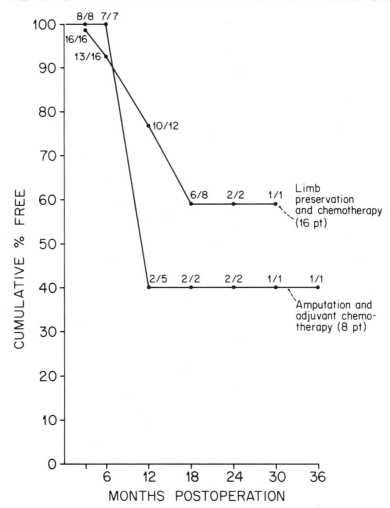

Figure 1. Cumulative percent of osteosarcoma patients free of recurrent disease over 2- to 36-months' follow-up. Proportions represent the number of patients who remained free of disease over those who were at risk of having a recurrence during the preceding time interval.

The high degree of necrosis observed in the tumor specimens after preoperative treatment with Adriamycin and radiation therapy is impressive—that an average of 86% of the tumor cells were destroyed attests to the efficacy of this approach. However, it is impossible to equate this histologic picture of cell death with the biologic potential for cellular regrowth. Therefore, preoperative treatment with Adriamycin and radiation therapy must be followed by en bloc excision of the primary tumor. No compromise relative to the extent of surgical excision should be considered.

The results of this and other studies indicate that complete excision of the involved bone and adjacent soft tissue is technically possible. Rarely do these tumors invade blood vessels or nerves; consequently, preservation of a viable, neurologically intact extremity can be achieved. Whether the cadaver allografts for bone replacement used in this study are superior to prosthetic implants remains to be seen. There is a question regarding the longevity of the allografts, particularly in the major weight-bearing areas, because of their tendency to fracture with time and to be reabsorbed by the host. However, we feel that continued use of these grafts is warranted by their availability and their potential for incorporation into the host as a viable structure.

We continue to be enthusiastic about the function of the allografts of the non-weight-bearing bones in the upper extremities. All patients have complete use of their hands and fingers, and therefore have much better function than they would with any prosthesis. However, before they can be compared with amputation or with metallic endoprostheses, the lower extremity allografts must be evaluated over longer follow-up periods.

The importance of continued, postoperative adjuvant chemotherapy cannot be overemphasized, because the effective control of subclinical distant metastatic disease will be the determining factor in the patient's survival. A longer period of observation obviously will be necessary to determine the ultimate fate of the salvaged limbs and, more importantly, the ultimate survival of these patients. Whether the favorable results achieved to date with adjuvant chemotherapy represent a cure of the disease or merely a delay in the appearance of metastases remains to be seen. Even if it does not effect cure, patients with malignant osteosarcoma are surviving longer than they did in the past. Since more limited surgery, combined with radiotherapy and chemotherapy, can preserve limbs with some degree of function, such treatment to improve the quality of these patients' lives must be given due consideration.

REFERENCES

1. Dahlin, D.C. and Coventry, M.B.: Osteogenic sarcoma: a study of 600 cases. *J Bone Joint Surg* 49A:101–196, 1967.

2. Cade, S.: Osteogenic sarcoma: a study based on 133 patients. *J R Coll Surg Edinb* 1:79–111, 1955.

3. Cortes, E.P., Holland, J.R., Wang, J.J. et al: Amputation and

Adriamycin in primary osteosarcoma. *N Engl J Med* 291:998–1000, 1974.

4. Jaffe, N.: Recent advances in the chemotherapy of metastatic osteosarcoma. *Cancer* 30:1627–1638, 1972.

5. Jaffe, N., Frei, E., III, Traggis, D. et al: Adjuvant methotrexate and citrovorum factor treatment of osteogenic sarcoma. *N Engl J Med* 291:994–997, 1974.

6. Jaffe, N. and Watts, H.G.: Multidrug chemotherapy in primary treatment of osteosarcomas: an editorial commentary. *J Bone Joint Surg* 58A:634–635, 1976.

7. Rosen, G., Suwansirikul, S., Kwan, C. et al: High-dose methotrexate with citrovorum factor rescue and Adriamycin in childhood osteosarcoma. *Cancer* 33:1151–1163, 1974.

8. Rosen, G., Murphy, M.L., Huvas, A.G. et al: Chemotherapy, en bloc resection, and prosthetic bone replacement in the treatment of osteogenic sarcoma. *Cancer* 37:1–11, 1976.

9. Isacoff, W.H., Townsend, C.M., Jr., Eilber, F.R. et al: High-dose methotrexate therapy of solid tumors: observations relating to clinical toxicity. *Med Pediatr Oncol* 2:319–325, 1976.

11 Surgical Treatment of Pulmonary Metastases from Osteosarcoma

Robert M. Filler, M.D.

Until recently the prognosis for those with osteosarcoma was dismal because most patients developed pulmonary metastases and died even though tumor at the primary site was completely eliminated. Surgical resection of pulmonary lesions was rarely feasible because metastases were almost always widely distributed. Chemotherapy and radiation therapy were also ineffective except in isolated cases.

The introduction of high-dose methotrexate and Adriamycin has radically improved the outlook for these patients.[1-7] Adjuvant chemotherapy programs have reduced the incidence of metastases, and even for those who develop lung lesions while on chemotherapy, the natural history of the disease appears to have been altered to such an extent that resection of these deposits is now possible in most cases. Thus, by combining surgery with intensive chemotherapy and radiotherapy in selected cases, many individuals with pulmonary metastases from osteosarcoma can now be saved.

CASE MATERIAL

Since 1972, 52 patients with newly diagnosed osteosarcoma and no pulmonary metastases have received adjuvant chemotherapy with high-dose methotrexate and other agents at the Sidney Farber Cancer Institute.[2-6] Sixteen of these 52 patients developed pulmonary metastases within 4 to 48 months from the time of initial diagnosis. In 10 of the 16, the lung lesions were removed surgically. During the same period, pulmonary metastases were resected in 6 other patients who were referred here when pulmonary metastases were first noted, 9 to 42 months after diagnosis. Three of these 6 patients had received no prior chemotherapy, 2 had been treated with one course of nitrogen mustard at the time of initial diagnosis. One additional patient had had a pulmonary resection. He was referred here with recurrent osteosarcoma of the skull with no pulmonary metastases. After the recurrence was resected, high-dose methotrexate was administered, but lung metastases became apparent 6 months later.

Of the 17 patients whose metastases were ultimately removed, the primary tumor was located in the lower extremity in 14, in the upper extremity in 2, and in the occiput in one. The primary tumor in the extremity had been treated by amputation in 14 patients. In 2 patients the involved limb was preserved and the primary tumor was treated by local en bloc resection after initial chemotherapy.[6] The age range of these patients was 6 to 19 years; 9 of the 17 were male.

SELECTION OF PATIENTS FOR SURGERY IN A MULTIDISCIPLINARY TREATMENT PROGRAM

Experience indicates that neither surgery, chemotherapy, nor radiation therapy alone can eliminate pulmonary metastases in the majority of patients and that a multidisciplinary approach will have greater success.[2-5] [7-11] The current treatment for pulmonary metastases is conducted in two phases. The objective in the first phase is to create a state in which clinically obvious disease is no longer apparent. In the second phase, treatment is continued to maintain this state. The schedule of multimodality treatment is adjusted for each patient and depends on the extent of disease, time elapsed from diagnosis, and previous treatment.[4]

Metastases which develop in patients who have never had prior chemotherapy are usually treated first by chemotherapy. Preoperative chemotherapy has the potential to minimize the surgical procedure, for in most cases some lesions disappear and others decrease in size. Presumably, micrometastases are also destroyed at this time. Although chemotherapy delays surgery, experience suggests that surgery has little value in untreated cases and in those in which chemotherapy has been ineffective. In general, several cycles of intensive chemotherapy are given for a period of four to six weeks.[3-5] [8]

When metastases appear soon after diagnosis, there is a greater likelihood that additional lesions will appear than there is when they develop later. Therefore, chemotherapy is continued for at least 9 months after initial diagnosis, as most metastases can be expected to occur in untreated patients by this time. Overt metastases are then resected in patients otherwise considered to be tumor-free after chemotherapy has arrested, or at least slowed, the progression of disease. In the current series, 6 of the 17 patients had either no chemotherapy or inadequate chemotherapy prior to the appearance of multiple pulmonary metastases. In 5 of these (cases 2, 9, 11, 14, and 17), pulmonary metastases were treated by intensive chemotherapy for 3 to 11 months before resection. In the sixth patient, the metastasis occupied half of the right thorax (Figure 1). Since chemotherapy and radiation therapy could not be expected to be very effective against a tumor of this size, the patient was treated first by surgery.

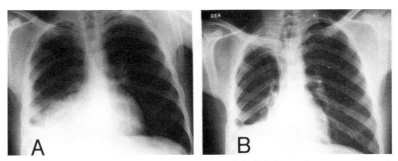

Figure 1. Case 1. Patient underwent amputation of the left femur for osteosarcoma in February 1974. **(A)** In October 1974, chest x-ray revealed a large metastasis which involved the right middle and lower lobe, the diaphragm, pericardium, and chest wall. All gross disease was resected and the patient received vincristine, methotrexate and citrovorum factor, and radiotherapy postoperatively. **(B)** Chest x-ray two years later, when chemotherapy was discontinued, showed no evidence of tumor. He remains alive and well 39 months after the original diagnosis.

The indications for surgery in patients whose metastases develop while they are on adjuvant chemotherapy are similar to those for patients who have never had chemotherapy (Table 1). Metastases which first appear after many months of chemotherapy are resected immediately after discovery, provided the patients are otherwise free of disease (cases 3, 4, 8, 15, and 16). However, development of multiple metastases soon after the start of adjuvant chemotherapy suggests that the natural behavior of the tumor has not been altered, and surgery should be deferred until progression of the lesions can be halted by other means. In our series of 52 patients who received adjuvant chemotherapy, 9 developed pulmonary metastases within six months of diagnosis. Lesions were multiple in all patients. In 3 cases (6, 10, and 12) the lesions did not progress with continued chemotherapy, and metastases were excised two to seven months later (Figure 2). In the other 6 patients, however, the lung lesions increased in size and number despite an intensive chemotherapy program, and surgery was deferred because it did not seem to offer any chance of improving survival.

Table 1
Indications for Surgical Treatment of Pulmonary Metastases

Immediate surgery*
  1. Bulk tumor unlikely to respond to chemotherapy
  2. Adequate prior chemotherapy
  3. Tumor developing after 9 months of adjuvant chemotherapy
  4. Late, isolated metastases

Delayed surgery†
  1. No prior chemotherapy
  2. Inadequate prior chemotherapy
  3. Metastases developing soon after diagnosis
  4. Metastases developing before completion of 9 months
     of adjuvant chemotherapy
  5. Stabilization and control of rapidly growing lesions achieved
     with chemotherapy

*Immediate surgery = surgery performed soon after appearance of metastases.
†Delayed surgery = surgery performed after an adequate trial of chemotherapy, generally four weekly courses of methotrexate and Adriamycin.

Pulmonary metastases do not develop in some patients until several years after initial diagnosis. This appears to be due either to the biologic behavior of the tumor or to tumor suppression by adjuvant chemotherapy (cases 5 and 6). In these cases metastases usually are few in number and are readily resectable. Thus, preoperative chemotherapy is omitted and potential microscopic deposits are treated postoperatively.

In deciding whether or not surgery is indicated, one must consider the number and size of the lesions to be removed. However, surgery is not contraindicated unless the amount of lung to be removed will produce pulmonary insufficiency. Similarly, surgery is not contraindicated in patients with metastatic lesions which involve the pleural space, pericardium, and diaphragm (Figure 1). The behavior of the tumor, rather than the number of metastases, is far more important in deciding operability. Patients with multiple

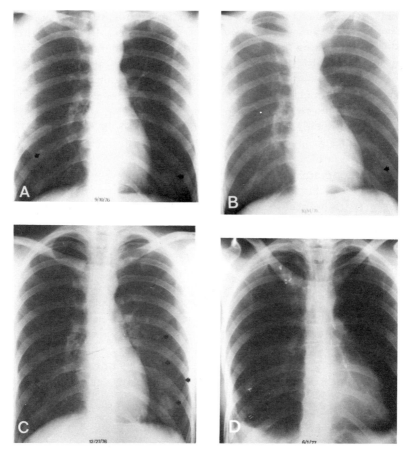

Figure 2. Case 6. Patient had osteosarcoma of the left femur, treated by en bloc local resection and insertion of a prosthesis to preserve the limb in July 1976 after two months of preoperative methotrexate. **(A)** In September, a pulmonary nodule was noted in each lung. **(B)** By October, one lesion had disappeared and the other had decreased in size on vincristine, methotrexate, and citrovorum factor. **(C)** By December, however, the nodules had enlarged and three new lesions had appeared. At thoracotomy in February 1977, three metastases in the left lower lobe were removed by lobectomy; two in the upper lobe were excised by wedge resection. The small lesion on the right increased in size, and at right thoracotomy in April 1977, two additional small nodules on the right were found. All were removed by wedge resection (Radiopaque clips indicate the sites of resection.) Chest x-ray in June **(D)** shows no residual disease, but it is too early to be certain of the long-term result.

lesions which have been stable for many months may have a better prognosis after surgery than will patients with one or two lesions which have appeared a month after diagnosis.

Chemotherapy is administered to almost all patients following surgery because, even after "complete" surgical resection, it is likely that residual microscopic tumor is still present. This residual tumor may be either at the site of resection, in the pleural cavity, in the lymphatics draining the local area, or at undetectable sites in other parts of the lung. This is particularly true of metastases treated within 18 months of diagnosis. The agents chosen and the duration of therapy depend on previous treatment.[4][8] The only patient in our series in whom chemotherapy was omitted was one who developed a single pulmonary metastasis 34 months after diagnosis and 10 months following completion of adjuvant chemotherapy (case 7). Microscopic study indicated that the solitary lesion was removed with adequate margins.

Postoperative radiation therapy is given when evidence at surgery or by histologic examination of the resected specimen suggests that the metastases have not been completely removed. Eleven of 17 patients in this series were treated with x-ray therapy. While osteosarcoma is not considered to be a radiosensitive tumor, radiotherapy has reduced, although not eradicated, primary lesions. It is reasonable to postulate that radiation treatment might be effective in helping to eradicate microscopic disease. The use of radiation therapy and chemotherapy concurrently was suggested by the observation that methotrexate produced recall erythema (similar to that produced by actinomycin D) in a previously irradiated area.[2] When a large volume of lung is treated, the radiation dose (1,500 rad in 12 days) is similar to that used for whole-lung treatment in children with Wilms' tumor.

SURGICAL MANAGEMENT

Preoperative Preparation

In most patients, the preparation for pulmonary resection need not be extensive. Since most patients have been on chemotherapy programs, it is essential that they have recovered fully from their last course of therapy. Mouth ulcers must be healed and intestinal function normal; white blood count, platelet count, and hematocrit should be in the normal range. Cardiac evaluation is necessary for all patients who have had Adriamycin therapy. Pulmonary function tests are not mandatory in patients who show no pulmonary symptoms and whose lungs have never been previously irradiated and do not contain other significant disease. A chest x-ray on the day prior to surgery is necessary to ascertain that no important changes have occurred from the time of previous diagnostic study. Instructions regarding postoperative physiotherapy are helpful before surgery, especially for the amputee whose mobility will be hampered by the operation.

Surgical Procedure

Since pulmonary metastases from osteosarcoma tend to be multiple, the principle of surgical treatment is to remove as much bulk tumor as possible and to minimize the loss of normal pulmonary tissue. Limited pulmonary resections are performed and chemotherapy and radiotherapy are relied upon to destroy residual microscopic disease. Except in those patients with massive pleural disease, only a small lateral thoracotomy is necessary; however, the incision should be large enough to allow exploration of all lobes. Often more lesions are found at surgery than were seen by x-ray. Tomograms can visualize lesions as small as 1.0 cm in diameter, but palpation can detect lesions one-fourth this size. Fortunately, osteosarcoma usually presents on the pleural surface of the lung, where it is relatively easy to find at surgery.

The majority of metastases can be removed by wedge resection. Many use a stapling instrument, but we have found it easier and more precise to outline the wedge of lung containing the metastases with two crushing Kelly clamps. The wedge is excised after a running suture has been placed through normal lung on the side of the clamps away from the tumor. It is useful to mark the site of surgery with metallic clips for future x-ray evaluation. Formal lobectomy is necessary when a single lobe is the site of many lesions or when the lobe cannot be salvaged because of the location and size of the metastases. In our series, lobectomy was performed in four cases (1, 6, 9, and 17).

Every attempt should be made to excise metastases which involve extrapulmonary thoracic sites such as the pericardium, diagphragm, and chest wall. These resections can be done safely and can produce gratifying results (Figure 1). In patients who present with bilateral metastases, thoracotomies are usually spaced a week or two apart. The surgical technique used for patients who have recurrent lesions is similar to that described for those undergoing their first procedure. However, recurrent lesions are more likely to involve the pleural space, and special care must be taken to avoid breaking into the tumor mass when dividing pleuro-pulmonary adhesions.

Since these young patients tolerate thoracotomy extremely well, postoperative chemotherapy and radiotherapy can be started within two weeks of surgery in the majority. Even though these modalities retard wound healing, no serious wound problems have occurred in our patients as a result of postoperative antitumor therapy.

RESULTS OF TREATMENT

In our series, a total of 38 thoracotomies were performed in 17 patients. In 12 of the 17, metastases were bilateral and lesions on each side required a separate operation. Six patients had additional resections because of recurrent pulmonary metastases (cases 4, 6, 11, 13, 16, and 17). One of these patients had three operations for recurrence (case 13), and another had two (case 16). In most patients, fewer than 5 metastatic lesions were resected; however, in four, 10 or more wedge resections were necessary. In one patient (case 10), 36 lesions were removed.

Surgical complications were remarkably few considering that most patients had had aggressive chemotherapy for at least several months before surgery. One patient (case 8) had a significant hemothorax, which was evacuated by surgery on the third postoperative day to free a trapped lung. A second patient (case 9) had a persistent air leak from the lung, which was treated successfully by continuous tube drainage for two weeks. A third patient (case 16) developed a localized empyema after excision of a recurrent tumor nodule. Tube thoracotomy was necessary for resolution. No other wound or pulmonary complications were noted. Most patients were able to leave the hospital within a week after surgery.

Eight of the 17 patients are currently well without evidence of disease (Table 2). Four have been followed for more than a year since surgery, and the other 4 have been operated on more recently. Two of these eight (cases 4 and 8) have had operations for recurrent disease which was noted within two months of surgery. In two others

Table 2
Clinical Data on Patients Alive and Well

Patient	Adjuvant Chemo- therapy*	Mos. from Diagnosis to Metastasis	No. of Thoracic Metastases		Other Thoracic Metastases	Preoperative Chemotherapy (months)
			Right Lung	Left Lung		
1	0	9	1	0	Diaphragm, pericardium, chest wall	0
2	2	42	3	2	Diaphragm	3
3	1	13	1	0		2
4	1	19	1	1		2.5
5	1	48	0	1		0
6	1	4	3	5		7
7	1	34	1	0		0
8	1	11	1	1		3

*0 = None; 1 = Vincristine, high-dose methotrexate, citrovorum rescue program; 2 = Adramycin; 3 = Nitrogen mustard
†+ = Excision of other thoracic lesions

Table 2 *(continued)*

Preoperative Chemotherapy (months)	Treatment of Metastases Surgery		Radiation Therapy	Postoperative Chemotherapy	Recurrence (months)	Additional Surgery	Months Since Last Surgery
	Right Lung	Left Lung					
0	2 Lobes + †		Yes	Yes	0	None	29
3	Wedge +	Wedge	Yes	Yes	0	None	12
2	Wedge		No	Yes	0	None	18
2.5	Wedge	Wedge	No	Yes	2	Wedge	12
0		Wedge	Yes	Yes	0	None	2
7	Wedge	Wedge & Lobe	No	Yes	0	None	3
0	Wedge		No	No	0	None	6
3	Wedge	Wedge	Yes	Yes	2	Wedge +	3

(cases 1 and 2) tumor which invaded the pleural cavity and extrapulmonary structures was excised when lesions in the lung were removed. Radiation therapy was used in 4 patients.

Five of the 17 patients have died, all as a result of their tumor; another 4 are living with disease (Table 3). In all 9, tumor recurred in the lung (usually within three months of surgery) despite postoperative chemotherapy in all and radiation therapy in 7. Reoperation in 4 also failed to control the progression of disease.

The survival curves for this group of patients and for that of a historical control group are shown in Figure 3. The median survival time for the control group was 9 months, and only 2 patients remained alive at 30 months. Survival among the current 17 patients was significantly better by both the double Wilcoxon and X^2 analyses $(P = 0.001)$.[12] Of greater importance is that almost half the patients rendered clinically free of disease continue to be well for from 2 to 29 months.

Comparison of patients free of disease (group 1) with those who have died or who are alive with disease (group 2) reveals major differences in both the number of metastases which appeared and the time from diagnosis which these lesions were detected. The average number of metastases in group 1 was 2.5, and six of the eight patients had 2 or less. The average interval from diagnosis to appearance of metastases in group 1 was 23 months (median: 19 months), but in group 2 the duration was only 11 months (median: 10 months). A comparison of other factors, such as the site of primary tumor, presence of pleural disease, use of chemotherapy, surgical technique, and use of radiation therapy, fails to reveal any obvious differences between the two groups.

Table 3
Clinical Data on Patients Either Alive with Disease or Dead

Patient	Adjuvant Chemo-therapy*	Mos. from Diagnosis to Metastasis	No. of Thoracic Metastases Right Lung	Left Lung	Other Thoracic Metastases	Preoperative Chemotherapy (mos.)	Treatment of Metastases Surgery Right Lung	Left Lung	Radiation Therapy	Postoperative Chemotherapy	Recurrence (months)	Additional Surgery	Months Since Last Surgery
9	0	16	1	2	Pleura, ribs	11	Lobe+†	Lobe	No	Yes	3	None	20‡
10	1	5	15	21	Pericardium	2	Wedge+	Wedge	Yes	Yes	3	None	4‡
11	0	10	5	5		5	Wedge	Wedge	Yes	Yes	2	Wedge	6‡
12	1	6	3	0		2	Wedge		Yes	Yes	3	None	11‡
13	1	16	8	10		3		Wedge	Yes	Yes	1,12,12	Wedge×3	7‡
14	2	10	6	4		6	Wedge	Wedge	Yes	Yes	1	None	15
15	1	16	1	1		2	Wedge	Wedge	No	Yes	8	None	19
16	1	14	3	1	Pleura	1	Wedge	Wedge+	Yes	Yes	3,15	Wedge×2	3
17	3	8	1	2		10	Lobe	Wedge	Yes	Yes	8	Wedge	6

*0 = None; 1 = Vincristine, high-dose methotrexate, citrovorum rescue program; 2 = Adramycin; 3 = Nitrogen mustard
†+ = Excision of other thoracic lesions
‡ = Dead

DISCUSSION

With current regimens of adjuvant chemotherapy, about 30% to 40% of patients with osteosarcoma may be expected to develop metastases. Even in those who develop metastases, there is evidence that chemotherapy has changed the natural behavior of the tumor. Thus, in patients given chemotherapy, the development of metastases is often delayed beyond 12 months from diagnosis, and in many patients only one or two lesions appear.

Even before effective chemotherapy was available, Martini et al advocated an aggressive surgical attack on pulmonary metastases.[9] In their series of 22 selected patients, many of whom had multiple nodules, 10 were alive 36 months after amputation and surgical removal of pulmonary metastases which developed after amputation.* The introduction of effective chemotherapy has resulted in the adoption of this aggressive surgical plan at a number of institutions.[4] [8] [10] Not only do more patients have isolated resectable disease than ever before, but now there is hope that chemotherapy will eradicate residual microscopic disease, which has been the cause of failure after surgery in the past. In the present series, 42% of the patients are alive without disease. Although the duration of follow-up in many is too short to be certain of a complete cure, their survival curves show a marked improvement over those of historical controls (Figure 3). Beattie et al and Kumar et al have reported similar findings.[8] [10]

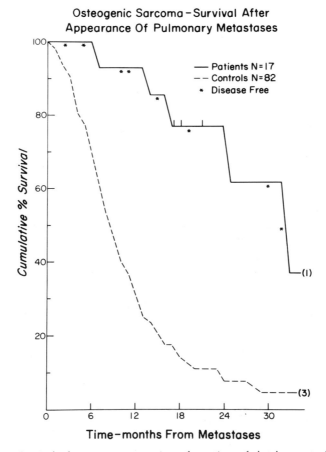

Osteogenic Sarcoma – Survival After Appearance Of Pulmonary Metastases

Figure 3. Survival of osteosarcoma patients from time of development of overt pulmonary metastases. Current series is compared to 82 historical controls.

---

*An update reports that 4 of the 10 have subsequently died of disease.[8]

Although chemotherapy can eliminate microfoci of cancer, evidence suggests that it cannot eradicate all the cells present in a macroscopic deposit. As a result, surgery is usually necessary to effect a complete cure. Current contraindications to surgery include the presence of tumor at extrathoracic sites, and rapidly growing pulmonary metastases which cannot be controlled by chemotherapy. Although the best results are obtained in patients with only one or two metastatic lesions, even those with more than ten should be given the benefit of surgery when no contraindications . exist. Similarly, an aggressive approach should be maintained for those with disease which recurs after initial thoractotomy, since our experience indicates that additional surgery can be curative.

In a previous study we assessed the role of pulmonary wedge resection for the treatment of lung metastases and concluded that lobectomy is a better operation for cancer.[11] However, this study also indicated that wedge resection could achieve local tumor control when combined with effective chemotherapy and radiation therapy, as in children with Wilms' tumor metastases. Because effective chemotherapy now appears to be available, wedge resection (which preserves more pulmonary tissue than lobectomy) is probably the procedure of choice for these metastases.

While major progress has been achieved in the treatment of all stages of osteosarcoma, the interpretation of results is limited to a framework of a maximum follow-up of four years. Therefore, attempts to extend and confirm our present observations are necessary. It is quite possible that modifications in our current approach will be necessary or that new modes of therapy will alter our approach completely.

REFERENCES

1. Cortes, E.P., Holland, J.F., Wang, J.J. et al: Amputation and Adriamycin in primary osteosarcoma. *N Engl J Med* 291:998–1000, 1974.

2. Jaffe, N., Farber, S., Traggis, D. et al: Favorable response of osteogenic sarcoma to high-dose methotrexate with citrovorum rescue and radiation therapy. *Cancer* 31:1367–1373, 1973.

3. Jaffe, N., Frei, E., III, Traggis, D. et al: Weekly high-dose methotrexate–citrovorum factor in osteogenic sarcoma: presurgical treatment of primary tumor and of overt pulmonary metastases. *Cancer* 39:45–50, 1977.

4. Jaffe, N., Traggis, D., Cassady, J.R. et al: Multidisciplinary treatment for macrometastatic osteogenic sarcoma. *Br Med J* 2:1039–1041, 1976.

5. Jaffe, N., Frei, E., III, Watts, H. et al: High-dose methotrexate in osteogenic sarcoma; a quinquennium of experience. *Cancer Treat Rep,* in press.

6. Jaffe, N., Watts, H., Fellows, K.E. et al: Local en bloc resection for limb preservation. *Cancer Treat Rep,* in press.

7. Rosen, G., Tan, C., Sanmaneechai, A. et al: The rationale for multiple drug chemotherapy in the treatment of osteogenic sarcoma. *Cancer* 35:936–945, 1975.

8. Beattie, E.J., Jr., Martini, N., and Rosen, G.: The management of pulmonary metastases in children with osteogenic sarcoma with surgical resection combined with chemotherapy. *Cancer* 35:618–621, 1975.

9. Martini, N., Huvos, A.G., Mike, V. et al: Multiple pulmonary resections in the treatment of osteogenic sarcoma. *Ann Thorac Surg* 12:271–297, 1971.

10. Kumar, A.P.M., Wrenn, E.L., Jr., Fleming, I.D. et al: Transmeduallary amputation and resection of metastases in combined therapy of osteosarcoma. *J Pediatr Surg* 12:427–435, 1977.

11. Ballantine, T.V.N., Wiseman, N.E., and Filler, R.M.: Assessment of pulmonary wedge resection for the treatment of lung metastases. *J Pediatr Surg* 10:671–676, 1975.

12. Gehan, E.A.: A generalized Wilcoxon test for comparing arbitrarily singly censored samples. *Biometrika* 52:203–223, 1965.

12 Radiation Therapy in Osteosarcoma

Ralph R. Weichselbaum, M.D.
J. Robert Cassady, M.D.

1. Management of the primary tumor
   a. Preoperative irradiation and delayed amputation
   b. Adjuvant chemotherapy
   c. Surgery
2. Management of metastatic disease: multimodality approach
   a. Radiation therapy

In malignant conditions, the efficacy of therapeutic strategies must be evaluated in light of their attendant complications. This principle, first elucidated by Holthusen, is of particular importance in analyzing the role of radiation therapy in osteosarcoma (Figure 1).[1] Although newer surgical techniques employing prostheses combined with chemotherapy may allow limb preservation in some patients, function continues to be suboptimal in many. In this chapter we will consider the utility of radiation therapy in the management of primary osteosarcoma with this concept in mind. Historical experience and current treatment policies will be reviewed, and the combined use of radiation therapy and chemotherapeutic regimens presently being investigated for treatment of metastatic disease will be discussed.

MANAGEMENT OF THE PRIMARY TUMOR

Preoperative Irradiation and Delayed Amputation

Because 80% of amputation patients 20 years ago experienced

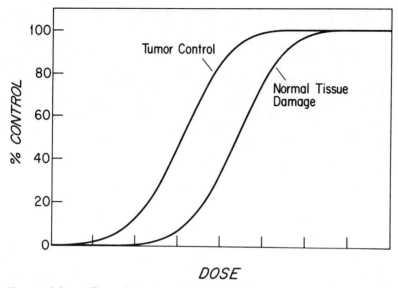

Figure 1. Schema illustrating concept of risk vs gain as described by Holthusen.[1] The effectiveness of tumor control is compared to normal tissue damage.

recurrence of metastatic disease in less than one year, Cade suggested a treatment program of preoperative irradiation and delayed amputation as an attempt to minimize unnecessary ablative surgical procedures.[2] Lee and McKenzie evaluated the efficacy of this approach in a large number of patients.[3] After initial evaluation for metastatic disease, usually by means of chest x-ray without tomography, patients were treated (with a 2-meV Van de Graaff machine) to a tumor dose of 7,000 to 8,000 rad during a period of seven to nine weeks (at 1,000 rad per week). Following a waiting period of four to six months, the patients were reevaluated, and those without evidence of metastatic disease underwent the prescribed amputation. Those who developed recurrent local disease prior to this time underwent surgical ablation. Radical extirpation was withheld whenever possible if tumor location made surgery unsuitable, if a potentially good response with continued good function were obtained, or if metastases developed. Of 92 patients who were treated according to this protocol, 70 died of disease, 2 were lost to follow-up, and 20 (21.8%) were alive without disease when last evaluated. Of the 20, seven had achieved control of the primary lesion without amputation. Apparently function was also maintained, although the quality of function is difficult to evaluate. In addition, the true incidence of local control is impossible to determine in those patients who developed metastases and did not undergo amputation.

Carceres and Zaharia have also used preoperative radiation therapy, consisting of 8,000 rad in 8 days or 12,000 rad in 12 days, in conjunction with amputation.[4] They found no particular advantage in this therapeutic regimen. Tudway has treated osteosarcoma patients with doses ranging from 5,500 to 8,000 rad, given over varying time spans.[5] Although 5 of 9 patients gained local control of tumor, fibrosis and disability were reported in 3 of these 5 patients, and thus only 2 of the 9 achieved apparently acceptable functional results.

These results have been corroborated by a retrospective study by Sweetnam et al and by our earlier experiences.[6] Jenkin and co-workers have reviewed the treatment of 42 osteosarcoma patients at the Princess Margaret Hospital.[7] A minimum dose of 4,200 rad had been given in 20 days using conventional radiation therapy techniques, and as much as 14,000 rad had been given some patients under hypoxic conditions. All of 27 patients treated with radical intent had suffered local recurrences with poor functional results. Patients treated under hypoxic conditions had experienced no advantage compared to those undergoing conventional radiation therapy.

Wright and Howard-Flanders, and Churchill-Davidson have suggested that anoxia may eliminate differential radiosensitivity between normal and tumor cells.[8] [9] In testing this, Suit treated 21 patients under local tissue hypoxia, delivering approximately 1,000 rad twice a week for a total tumor dose of 8,000 to 14,000 rad in 23 to 32 days.[10] Eleven patients with osteosarcoma of the distal femur or proximal tibia were treated in this fashion. Subsequent biopsies in 7 of these patients demonstrated local recurrences in 5. Radiation necrosis also developed in 5 of 6 patients in whom the total tourniquet time was 30 minutes per session. Thus, not only did hypoxia not yield the expected therapeutic advantages, but severe normal tissue sequelae developed.

Adjuvant Chemotherapy

In view of the documented incidences of local failure, conventional radiation therapy directed at the primary tumor is no longer tenable. Such potentially uncontrolled primary disease poses a major threat of continuous seeding of tumor cells, as well as possible development of resistance to effective chemotherapy, leading, ultimately, to widespread metastasis and death.

The observation by Jaffe et al and Cortes et al that metastatic osteosarcoma can respond to chemotherapy has led to the use of systemic adjuvant therapy for eradication of micrometastases.[11] [12]

These and other chemotherapeutic regimens have been incorporated into modern treatment programs and are used in conjunction with radiation therapy for treatment of the primary lesion when surgery is infeasible or impossible — either because a lesion is too extensive for amputation; because there are axial skeleton lesions; or because amputation is rejected. One such regimen utilizes radiation therapy and concurrent administration of radiopotentiating agents such as 5-bromodeoxyuridine (BUDR) or high-dose methotrexate in selected patients. This approach is under investigation (particularly for the treatment of inoperable tumors) at The Children's Hospital at Stanford (using BUDR) and in our clinics (using high-dose methotrexate). Goffinet et al have administered large fractions (600 rad) 48 hours after pulse BUDR at five-day intervals.[13] Initially, toxicity to normal tissue was excessive, but improved techniques in more recently treated patients have resulted in continued satisfactory local control. The preliminary trials in these patients will determine the feasibility of this approach for improving function.

Surgery

It must be stressed that surgical treatment of the primary tumor (amputation or, when feasible, resection) is considered the treatment of choice. We recommend primary radiation therapy only for older patients who refuse surgical procedures or for those in whom the tumor is located in an anatomic position where surgery is not possible. In extremity lesions, radiation therapy is delivered to the entire bone to a total dose of approximately 4,000 rad, giving 200 rad per fraction five days a week. In addition, "cone-down" treatment is given, so the original volume of tumor receives a total dose of 6,600 to 7,000 rad. In all cases, a generous strip of soft tissue must be spared for retention of adequate lymphatic circulation. Radiation therapy should be accompanied by administration of high-dose methotrexate and citrovorum factor "rescue." Suitable downward adjustments in radiation dosage should be made when radiopotentiating drugs such as Adriamycin or BUDR are used.

In lesions of the axial skeleton, the volume of tissue treated must be individualized. However, the suggested minimum total tumor dose is 6,600 to 7,000 rad, given in fractions of 200 rad daily for five days a week.

The preferred treatment for limb preservation would probably be preoperative chemotherapy with en bloc resection of tumor and prosthetic bone replacement, which has been described by Rosen et al and by Jaffe et al with encouraging preliminary results.[14] [15] However, this course is not adopted for lower extremity lesions if the patient has not attained mature growth, because there will be disproportionate growth of the contralateral limb. Immature growth status is also a contraindication to radiation therapy, which, while preserving the limb, may cause growth arrest and adversely affect limb function.

MANAGEMENT OF METASTATIC DISEASE: MULTIMODALITY APPROACH

Despite adjuvant therapy, nearly half of the patients with osteosarcoma may present with or develop metastatic disease. Prophylactic lung irradiation, alone or in combination with chemotherapeutic agents not known to be effective in osteosarcoma has shown no decided advantage in preventing the development of metastases.[16] When metastases develop, surgery, radiation therapy, and chemotherapy—alone or in combination—have been utilized. The median survival time of patients with untreated metastatic disease is less than four months, and 90% of all such patients die within one year.[17]

Radiation Therapy

While a combination of surgery and chemotherapy has been used to eradicate pulmonary metastases, recurrences are still possible after such treatment.[18] [19] In an attempt to reduce this incidence, Weichselbaum et al employed an aggressive, multi-modality approach for treatment of metastatic pulmonary osteosarcoma which included radiation therapy, chemotherapy, and surgery.[20] In general, whole-lung irradiation (1,500 rad given in ten fractions during two weeks) was employed concurrently with weekly high-dose methotrexate. In addition, cone-down radiation therapy doses varying between 2,000 and 4,000 rad (depending on the total tumor volume) were administered to areas of known or probable microscopic residual disease. Approximately 80% of the areas of high risk received a radiotherapy dose of 2,000 rad. (A "high-risk" area is defined as a site of previous excision of gross disease.) Following radiation therapy, adjuvant chemotherapy was continued. In this experience, control of pulmonary osteosarcoma was achieved after gross disease resection and delivery of a high cone-down dose to a small volume.

Although local control was initially achieved in the patients who developed metastases while receiving adjuvant chemotherapy, the majority ultimately developed disease in extrapulmonary sites, often in other bones. While eventual death in this subgroup of patients appears likely, the duration of survival has been increased significantly. Localized extrapulmonary metastasis may be palliated with relatively high doses of radiation (3,500 to 4,500 rad) delivered at accelerated fractionation schemes (250 to 300 rad per fraction, depending upon the volume to be treated). Cord compression may require emergency laminectomy as well as radiation therapy.

The need for "prophylactic" lung irradiation in combination with systemic chemotherapy, including high-dose methotrexate, is speculative. Currently, 30% to 40% of patients relapse despite adjuvant chemotherapy, principally because of lung metastases. Frei, using extrapolations from laboratory and clinical models, has calculated that an average of 10^9 tumor cells must be present in the lung before they become clinically apparent.* Using kinetic models, he suggests that currently employed adjuvant chemotherapeutic approaches can control from 10^5 to 10^6 cells. Patients with tumor cell burdens greater than this, which are principally located in the lungs, represent that patient group which currently fails despite adjuvant therapy. It is possible, however, that the addition of radiation therapy to a potentially localized tumor area in a lung might further reduce the malignant cell burden and permit cure in a large fraction of patients. Despite limited pulmonary radiation tolerance, there is abundant experimental and clinical evidence that radiation is effective in controlling microscopic disease.[21][22] Should these speculations prove valid, even a limited additional cell kill (10^3 to 10^4 cells) might substantially improve current results.

In summary, radiation therapy currently has a limited but definite role in the treatment of primary and metastatic osteosarcoma. It is possible that effective adjuvant chemotherapy in combination with radiation therapy may prove to be advantageous and that a broader role may thereby be defined for radiation therapy in this disease.[23]

REFERENCES

1. Holthusen, H.: Erfahrungen über die vertraglich keitsgrenze für Röntgenstrahlen und deren Nutzanwendung zur Verhütung von Schaden. *Strahlentherapie* 57:254, 1936.

2. Cade, S.: Editorial. *Ann R Coll Surg Engl* 9:211, 1955.

3. Lee, S.E. and MacKenzie, D.H.: Osteosarcoma. *Br J Surg* 51:252–274, 1964.

4. Carceres, E. and Zaharia, M.: Massive preoperative radiation therapy in the treatment of osteogenic sarcoma. *Cancer* 30:634–638. 1972.

---

*E. Frei 1977: personal communication.

5. Tudway, R.D.: Radiotherapy for osteogenic sarcoma. *J Bone Joint Surg* 43B:61–67, 1961.

6. Sweetnam, R., Knowleden, J., and Seddon, H.: Bone sarcoma: treatment by irradiation and amputation or a combination of the two. *Br Med J* 2:363–367, 1971.

7. Jenkin, R.D.T., Allt, W.E.C., and Fitzpatrick, P.J.: Osteosarcoma and assessment of management, with particular reference to primary irradiation with selective delayed amputation. *Cancer* 30:393–400, 1972.

8. Wright, E.A. and Howard-Flanders, P.: The influence of oxygen on the radio-sensitivity of mammalian tissues. *Acta Radiol* 48:26–32, 1957.

9. Churchill-Davidson, I.: The oxygen effect in radiotherapy. In Raven, W.R., (ed): *Cancer Progress*, Vol. 2. Butterworth & Co., London, 1960, pp 164–179.

10. Suit, H.D.: Radiation therapy given under conditions of local tissue hypoxia for bone and soft tissue sarcoma. In M.D. Anderson Hospital: *Tumors of Bone and Soft Tissue.* Year Book Medical Publishers, Inc., Chicago, 1965, pp 143–163.

11. Jaffe, N., Frei, E., Traggis, D. et al: Adjuvant methotrexate and citrovorum factor treatment of osteogenic sarcoma. *N Engl J Med* 291:994–997, 1974.

12. Cortes, E.P., Holland, J.F., Wang, J.J. et al: Amputation and Adriamycin in primary osteosarcoma. *N Engl J Med* 291:998–1000, 1974.

13. Goffinet, D.R., Kaplan, H.S., Donaldson, S.S. et al: Combined radiosensitizer infusion and irradiation of osteogenic sarcomas. *Radiology* 117:211–214, 1975.

14. Rosen, G., Murphy, M.L., Huvos, A.G. et al: Chemotherapy, en bloc resection, and prosthetic bone replacement in the treatment of osteogenic sarcoma. *Cancer* 37:1–11, 1976.

15. Jaffe, N., Frei, E., III, Traggis, D. et al: Weekly high-dose methotrexate-citrovorum factor in osteogenic sarcoma. Presurgical treatment of primary tumor and of overt pulmonary metastases. *Cancer* 39:45–50, 1977.

16. Rab, T.G., Ivins, J.C., Childs, D.C. et al: Elective whole-lung irradiation in the treatment of osteogenic sarcoma. *Cancer* 38:939–942, 1976.

17. Marcove, R.C., Mike, V., Hajek, J.V. et al: Osteogenic sarcoma under the age of 21: a review of 145 operative cases. *J Bone Joint Surg* 52A:411–423, 1974.

18. Martini, N., Huvos, A., Mike, V. et al: Multiple pulmonary resections in the treatment of osteogenic sarcoma. *Ann Thorac Surg* 12:271–280, 1971.

19. Beattie, E.J., Martini, N., and Rosen, R.: The management of pulmonary metastasis in children with osteogenic sarcoma with surgical resection combined with chemotherapy. *Cancer* 35:618–621, 1975.

20. Weichselbaum, R.R., Cassady, J.R., Jaffe, N. et al: Preliminary results of aggressive multimodality therapy for metastatic osteosarcoma. *Cancer* 40:78–83, 1977.

21. Shipley, W.V., Stanley, J.A., and Steel, G.G.: Tumor size dependency in the radiation response of the Lewis lung carcinoma. *Cancer Res* 35:2488–2493, 1975.

22. Fletcher, G.I.: *Textbook of Radiotherapy*. Lea & Febiger, Philadelphia, 1973.

23. Caldwell, W.L.: Elective whole-lung irradiation. *Radiology* 120:659–666, 1976.

13 Radiation Therapy in Ewing's Sarcoma

J. Robert Cassady, M.D.

Radiation therapy as the primary treatment for Ewing's sarcoma offers the possibility of tumor control of the affected bone together with preservation of function. As such, it is generally acknowledged to be the primary treatment of choice for the majority of patients with this aggressive malignancy.[1-5] Exacting radiation therapy technique is necessary to obtain the highest degree of tumor control possible while keeping the incidence and severity of complications to a minimum. The concurrent use of several chemotherapeutic agents, necessary for systemic control of micrometastases (which are thought to be present in most patients), further complicates the task of the radiation oncologist.[6]

RADIATION THERAPY TECHNIQUE

Ewing's sarcoma arises most often in the diaphyseal region of a bone and tends to originate in the medullary portion. Transmedullary spread throughout the affected bone occurs frequently, and therefore the entire bone is irradiated during a major portion of the treatment course. In addition, because of the extensive degree of soft tissue invasion, the field initially irradiated includes major portions of the soft tissues of the affected extremity or body region. However, throughout the course of radiation therapy, care must be taken to maintain a significant strip of nonirradiated skin and subcutaneous tissues. These should total at least 1.5 to 2.0 cm in order to prevent late lymphedema and constrictive fibrosis. Since vascular and lymphatic channels are most abundant in the medial portion of both the upper arm and upper leg, this nonirradiated strip should be located medially when disease extent permits. If possible, the irradiated extremity should be maintained in the same position and immobilized in an identical fashion for both the initial and for subsequent, "cone-down" fields. This precaution will ensure that the nonirradiated skin and subcutaneous tissue remain intact.

Although no information is available on any treatment series in which routine lymph node biopsy has been performed, lymph node involvement with Ewing's sarcoma is not frequently noted clinically. Thus, we do not perform routine irradiation of clinically uninvolved primary nodal sites. However, some primary nodes are automatically irradiated when bones such as the femur or innominate are treated. We have seen no patients with primary relapse in the meninges and/or brain. A number of other recently reported series of patients treated with primary radiation therapy and multiagent systemic chemotherapy without central nervous system (CNS) prophylactic treatment also fail to demonstrate a substantial primary CNS relapse rate.[2,3,5,7,8] Therefore, although some advocated this measure, we do not treat patients with prophylactic neuraxis irradiation.[4,9]

The initial treatment dose consists of 4,000 to 4,500 rad over 28 to 30 days, with daily fractions of 180 to 200 rad given five times a week. Successive cone-down fields are then introduced for an additional 1,500 to 1,800 rad, for a total minimum tumor dose of 5,500 to 5,800 rad given over approximately six to seven weeks. When possible, all fields should be treated daily in order to minimize adverse radiation effects on normal tissues and to provide daily tumor dose homogeneity. No dose adjustment is made on the basis of patient age at initiation of therapy.

Megavoltage irradiation is essential, and a linear accelerator has technical advantages—particularly that of sharpness of beam edge—over cobalt 60 equipment. Other technical details include immobilization techniques, such as individually constructed casts, to ensure reproducibility in daily treatment (Figure 1). Major differences in tissue thickness between the distal and proximal or medial and lateral portions of an extremity or body part often necessitate use of a three-dimensional compensator and/or wedge filter to achieve homogeneity of dose. When tumor invasion into skin or subcutaneous tissue occurs, appropriate bolus is necessary with megavoltage photon energies. Bolus of the biopsy incision site may also be required.

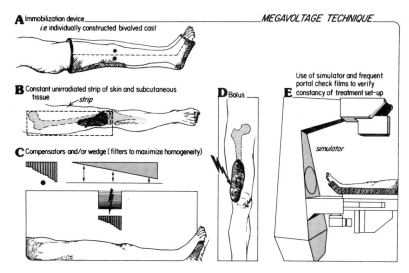

Figure 1. Schematic diagram illustrating several technical aspects of radiation therapy technique necessary to ensure optimum results. These techniques include: (a)immobilization device; (b)constant unirradiated strip of skin and subcutaneous tissue; (c)compensators and/or wedge (filters); (d)bolus; and (e)use of simulator and frequent portal check films to verify constancy of treatment set-up.

CONCURRENT CHEMOTHERAPY

In patients who do not present with evident metastatic disease, radiation therapy to the primary lesion is administered concurrently with chemotherapy. In our clinics chemotherapy usually includes vincristine, actinomycin D, and cyclophosphamide (see Chapter 6).[5] Cyclophosphamide may be omitted initially in these patients to avoid prolonged myelosuppression with its attendant, possibly significant alteration in radiation fractionation. It is also omitted when the bladder is included in the portal of radiation. Potentiation of radiation effect by actinomycin D may also necessitate short treatment breaks for cutaneous or mucosal reactions. This is particularly true when the gastrointestinal tract is involved. Actinomycin D may therefore be omitted initially if large areas of bowel are included in the radiation portal.

Patients who present with metastatic disease are treated initially with unmodified chemotherapy. This usually consists of vincristine, actinomycin D, cyclophosphamide, and Adriamycin administered in various combinations.[2][3][5][7] Depending on the site of primary lesion and any anticipated reactions due to combined use of radiation therapy and chemotherapy, primary radiation therapy may either be given concurrently with chemotherapy or it may be administered four to six weeks later. No major alterations in radiation therapy dose or technique for the primary lesion are introduced unless required by the patient's clinical status. Attempting to consolidate the effects of primary chemotherapy by irradiating the sites of metastatic (or prior metastatic) disease in selected patients may also be useful.[5]

CASE MATERIAL

From January 1971 to June 1976 we treated 20 patients with Ewing's sarcoma with radiation therapy (7 other patients were seen, but they are excluded from discussion here because primary radiation therapy was not delivered at our center). Eight of the 20 presented with evidence of distant metastatic disease (4 each to lung and to bone) as demonstrated roentgenographically or by isotopic scan. In addition, one patient demonstrated apparent simultaneous double primary lesions (in the right ulna and humerus) and another had a spinal lesion with contiguous extension to multiple bones and soft tissue (Table 1). Thus, only 10 of the 20 presented with disease limited to the bone of origin and the adjacent soft tissues (Table 2). Actuarial survival for all patients and for this latter, favorable group is shown in Figure 2. Clinical and treatment data for, and current status of, these patients are shown in Table 3. No patient presenting with distant metastatic disease has shown long-term disease-free survival (i.e., survival for more than two years).

COMPLICATIONS

Complications of high-dose radiation therapy in combination with chemotherapy can be divided into three categories: (1) acute: those occurring during or shortly after the period of irradiation; (2) delayed: complications occurring several weeks after irradiation; and (3) chronic: complications occurring months to years later.

Acute complications include erythema and, on very rare occasions, moist desquamation, which usually appears 14 to 21 days after initiation of therapy, at the peak period of interaction between irradiated tissues and actinomycin D. Patients with pelvic or lumbosacral lesions often develop nausea, vomiting, or diarrhea during

Table 1
Clinical Data on Ten Cases of Metastatic Ewing's Sarcoma

Primary Tumor Site	No. of Patients	Relapse Site			Disease-Free Survival for More Than Two Years
		No Remission	Lung	Other Bone	
Femur	2		1	1	
Humerus and Ulna*	1				1
Pelvis	1		1		
Spine†	2		1		1
Clavicle	1		1		
Rib	3	1	2		
Total	10	1	6	1	2

*Double primary lesions
†These two patients were treated with vincristine, Adriamycin, and cyclophosphamide followed by "pulse" doses of vincristine, actinomycin D, and cyclophosphamide.

Table 2
Clinical Data on Ten Cases of Nonmetastatic Ewing's Sarcoma

Primary Tumor Site	No. of Patients	Relapse Site			Disease-Free for More Than Two Years
		Local	Lung	Bone	
Femur	3	1			2
Ulna	1				1
Fibula	1				1
Pelvis	3		1	1	1
Spine	1				1
Rib	1				1
Total	10	1	1	1	7

irradiation. These are usually well controlled with appropriate therapy. Sequential radiographs of the affected bone during the course of treatment often show an apparent extension of the lesion despite subjective improvement or objective decrease in soft tissue mass. We have seen no instances of confirmed tumor growth during irradiation, and we surmise that any apparent extension indicates subclinical extension of tumor which was present at initiation of treatment and which becomes evident upon tumor reduction and treatment-related bone demineralization.

Another potentially catastrophic acute complication is pathologic fracture of the affected bone secondary to extensive bone destruction—from either tumor or, more frequently, and excessively large or poorly placed biopsy site (Figure 3). Accordingly,

196

biopsy should be just sufficient to establish the presence and type of malignancy. When such a fracture occurs, however, mechanical fixation with a metallic device is necessary to permit healing (Figure 4). Following surgical fixation, radiation therapy should be reinstated as soon as possible.

Delayed Recall of radiation reaction, especially of the skin, frequently occurs with the first postirradiation course of chemotherapy, when agents such as actinomycin D or Adriamycin, which potentiate radiation effects, are used. Approximately six to eight weeks following completion of radiation therapy, erythema, increased skin temperature, and edema of the irradiated skin and subcutaneous tissue are frequently seen, occasionally in association with local tenderness. This reaction usually lasts for one to three

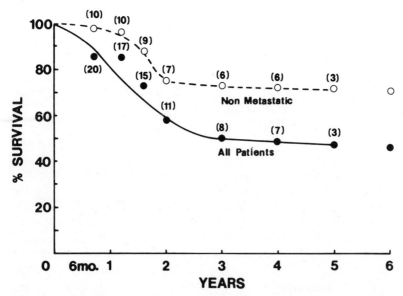

Figure 2. Actuarial survival curves for all patients and for those with limited disease (Tables 1 and 2). Numbers in parentheses represent numbers of patients; the open and closed circles at 6 years represent a single patient.

weeks. Although clearly related to irradiation, it is not always associated with chemotherapy and its exact pathogenesis is unknown.

Chronic Late complications may include significant subcutaneous fibrosis and growth arrest of both the irradiated bone and adjacent muscle. It is evident that the magnitude of these changes relates not only to technical details of irradiation and chemotherapy but also to the area treated and to the age and size (relative to dose received) of the patient. If subcutaneous fibrosis is severe, contractures of the treated extremity may occur.

Pathologic fractures are also not uncommon, especially in the 18- to 24-month post-radiation-treatment period, while chemotherapy is being administered.[10] Two of our patients with irradiated extremities developed this complication, which almost invariably occurs at the tumor biopsy site. Demineralization and the decreased ability to heal associated with combination therapy make

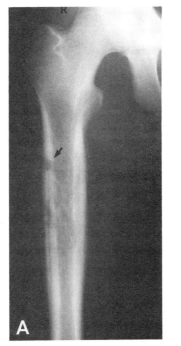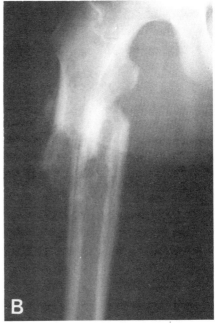

Figure 3. Illustration of a pathologic fracture occurring during treatment. **(A)** Note lucency from biopsy site (arrow) and relationship of this further-weakened area to subsequent fracture **(B)** Patient required mechanical fixation of fracture site and is surviving free of disease.

Table 3
Clinical and Treatment Data on Twenty Patients with Ewing's Sarcoma Treated with Radiation Therapy and Chemotherapy

Patient	Sex	Age (years)	Tumor Site	Metastases	Date of Presentation	Total Radiation Dose/Days(d)	X-ray Complications	Function	Local Control*	Relapse	Current Status[†]
1	M	6¹¹⁄₁₂	Femur	None	12/71	5,525 rad 40d	Mild subcutaneous fibrosis, moderate shortening	Excellent	+	None	NED[†]
2	M	9	Fibula	None	12/71	5,600 rad 43d	Pathologic fracture 9/72, mild shortening	Excellent	+	None	NED
3	M	11⁵⁄₁₂	Femur	None	12/71	5,600 rad 48d	Pathologic fracture, mild subcutaneous fibrosis and shortening	Excellent	+	None	NED
4	M	12	Ulna	None	1/74	5,600 rad 41d	None	Excellent	+	None	NED
5	M	7	Femur	None	5/73	5,500 rad 40d	Moderate shortening	Excellent until recurrence	–	Local, lung	Alive with tumor
6	M	7	Ilium	None	5/71	5,000 rad 36d	None	Excellent	+	Bone, lung	Dead 3/73
7	M	8	Rib	None	4/73	5,600 rad 40d	None	Excellent	+	None	NED
8	F	15	Lumbar spine	None	11/75	5,400 rad 41d	None	Excellent	+	None	NED
9	F	9	Right humerus, ulna	? Double primary	4/76	5,800 rad 52d	Moderate edema of extremity, marked subcutaneous fibrosis and contracture	Poor	+	None	NED
10	M	14	Ilium, pubis	None	6/76	6,000 rad 50d	Mild subcutaneous fibrosis	Excellent	+	None	NED

11	F	12	Sacrum	Massive soft tissue extension to left spine	7/75	5,474 rad 50d	None	Excellent	+	None	NED
12	M	12	Ilium	None	9/73	5,800 rad 47d	None	Excellent	+	Lung	Dead 1/75
13	M	16	Ilium, sacrum	Bone (skull), lung	1/76	5,500 rad 52d	Mild subcutaneous fibrosis, mild contracture	Good	+	Lung, skull	Alive with tumor
14	M	8	Femur, ischium, para-aortic nodes	Ilium	11/74	5,800 rad 45d	None	Good	+	Lung	Dead 1/75
15	M	17	Rib	Pleura, soft tissue	1/73	5,475 rad 49d	None	Excellent	Marginal recurrence in pleura	Progression of metastases	Dead
16	M	11	Tibia	Bone	10/72	6,000 rad 41d	Persistent ulcer post biopsy	Good until biopsy	+	Lung	Dead 12/74
17	M	13	Femur	Lung	9/72	6,700 rad 56d	Flexion contracture, marked fibrosis	Poor	+	Progression of lung metastases	Dead 10/73
18	M	7	Clavicle	Lung	8/71	5,000 rad 51d	None	Excellent	+	Progression of lung metastases	Dead 5/74
19	F	12	Rib	Lung, pleura	2/73	5,483 rad 43d	Pulmonary function decrease	Good	+	Lung metastases	Alive with tumor
20	F	10	Rib	Bone, pleura	2/71	Palliative	None	Pain relief	No attempt at primary control	Progression of metastatic disease	Dead 7/71

*+ = control achieved; − = control not achieved
†NED = No evidence of disease

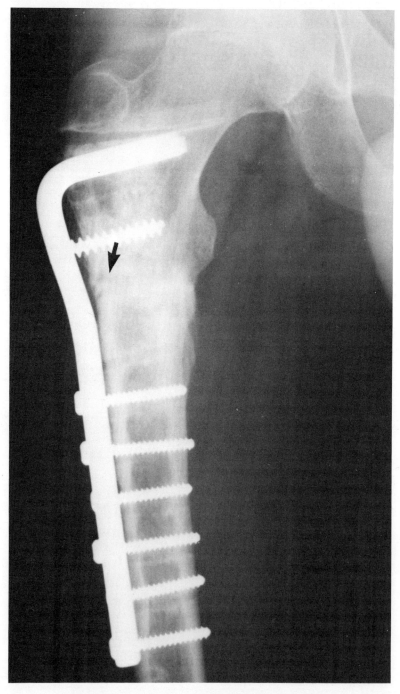

Figure 4. Metallic fixation of pathologic fracture (arrow).

this a more common chronic complication, and one more difficult to treat, although conservative therapy permitted healing in our patients. When a nonirradiated strip of skin and subcutaneous tissue has been maintained, significant late extremity edema has not been seen.

Finally, secondary neoplasms within the irradiated field (not observed to date in these patients) represent a potential, major late complication.[11] Despite these possible ill effects, it must be remembered that the great majority of patients with localized disease who are so treated survive with excellent function and local control.

CURRENT RECOMMENDATIONS

Our experiences with Ewing's sarcoma demonstrate that the optimum therapeutic approach strives for an acceptable balance between tumor control (both local and systemic) and satisfactory function. As function is of considerable importance, radiation therapy will most often be utilized for control of the primary lesion (Figure 5). Radiation doses above 5,500 to 6,000 rad administered in conjunction with chemotherapeutic regimens have not produced convincing evidence of improved local control rates, which suggests that the plateau of the sigmoid dose-response curve has been reached at this dosage level.[3] However, functional morbidity increases markedly with radiation doses above 6,000 rad.[7][12] Therefore, as with most tumors, there is a narrow range between the optimum and an excessive radiation dose. In view of this narrow range, it is essential that every technique be utilized to ensure maximum homogeneity of dose in the tumor volume. Without such care, the complication rate will be unacceptable in relation to any improvement in local control.

Functional considerations also may lead to surgery as the primary therapy of choice in some (albeit a minority of) patients. Patients with lower extremity lesions who have no apparent metastases and who are extremely young (less than six years) at the time of presentation may particularly benefit from initial surgical management, as irradiation causes total or considerable growth arrest of the treated bone, with subsequent marked leg-length discrepancy. (However, amputation at this early age is not without significant difficulties.) Surgical treatment of primary lesions arising in bones with limited significance (rib, clavicle, fibula) may also permit smaller radiation fields to be used, with less associated morbidity. In the very exceptional patient with no soft tissue extension, withholding radiation therapy following adequate surgery may be possible.

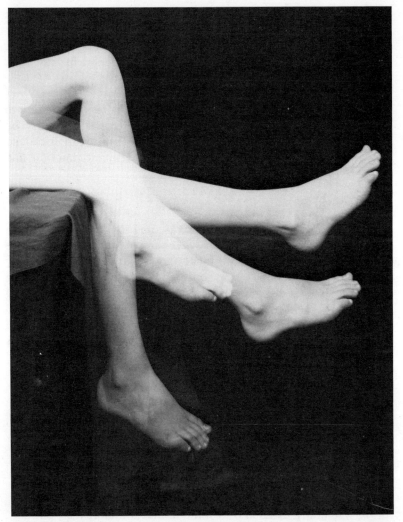

Figure 5. Range of motion in continuously disease-free 15-year-old patient treated six years previously (5,600 rad given in 28 fractions during 43 days) for fibula primary. Patient has full range of motion and minimal leg-length discrepancy and pursues normal activities.

The importance of adjuvant chemotherapy cannot be overemphasized. Prior to the routine employment of chemotherapy it was the exceptional patient who did not succumb to metastatic disease, despite local control.[6] The addition of chemotherapeutic regimens has undoubtedly improved survival and has almost certainly increased the proportion of cured patients.[4] However, the adjuvant regimen—the proper schedule and dosage of such agents in combination with irradiation—will be influenced by the site of the lesion. Most, if not all, of the agents used in currently effective regimens may be associated with toxicities, some of which may also mimic radiation effects.[12] In addition, significant potentiation of radiation effect also occurs. In the patient with no detectable metastatic disease, radiation therapy assumes primary importance, and chemotherapy, although administered concurrently, should be modified appropriately. Conversely, for the patient who presents with metastatic disease, chemotherapy assumes greater importance, and radiation schedules should be adjusted to permit maximum utilization of these agents.

Finally, careful follow-up of the patient by the radiation oncologist is essential. This follow-up must include collaboration with the orthopedic surgeon for optimum functional results. Through such efforts, appropriate, active physiotherapy to reduce contractures, and orthopedic management of posttreatment leg-length discrepancy and other, related problems will be ensured. In addition, treatment-related complications such as pathologic fracture, infection, and, most importantly, local recurrence of tumor will be detected if such a follow-up procedure is practiced.

With optimum management, over half of the patients with Ewing's sarcoma who present without metastases may today achieve tumor control and excellent function. This represents a major achievement for multimodality therapy.

REFERENCES

1. Boyer, C.W., Jr., Brickner, T.J., Jr., and Perry, R.H.: Ewing's sarcoma: case against surgery. Cancer 20:1602–1606, 1967.

2. Hustu, H.O., Pinkel, D., and Pratt, C.B.: Treatment of clinically localized Ewing's sarcoma with radiotherapy and combination chemotherapy. Cancer 30:1522–1527, 1972.

3. Fernandez, C.H., Lindberg, R.D., Sutow, W.W. et al: Localized Ewing's sarcoma: treatment and results. Cancer 34:143–148, 1974.

4. Pomeroy, T.C. and Johnson, R.E.: Combined modality therapy of Ewing's sarcoma. Cancer 35:36–47, 1975.

5. Jaffe, N., Traggis, D., Sallan, S. et al: Improved outlook for Ewing's sarcoma with combination chemotherapy and radiation therapy. Cancer 38:1925–1930, 1976.

6. Falk, S. and Alpert, M.: Five-year survival of patients with Ewings' sarcoma. Surg Gynecol Obstet 124:319–324, 1967.

7. Rosen, G., Wollner, N., Tan, C. et al: Disease-free survival in children with Ewing's sarcoma treated with radiation therapy and adjuvant four-drug sequential chemotherapy. Cancer 33:384–393, 1974.

8. Jenkin, R.D.T., Rider, W.D., and Sonley, M.J.: Ewing's sarcoma. *Int J Radiat Oncol Biol Phys* 1:407–413, 1976.

9. Marsa, G.W. and Johnson, R.J.: Altered pattern of metastasis following treatment of Ewing's sarcoma with radiotherapy and adjuvant chemotherapy. *Cancer* 27:1051–1054, 1971.

10. Bonarigo, B.C. and Rubin, P.: Non-union of pathologic fracture after radiation therapy. *Radiology* 88:889–898, 1967.

11. Li, F.P., Cassady, J.R., and Jaffe, N.: Risk of second tumors in survivors of childhood cancer. *Cancer* 35:1230–1235, 1975.

12. Tefft, M., Lattin, P.B., Jereb, B. et al: Treatment of rhabdomyosarcoma and Ewing's sarcoma of childhood. Acute and late effects on normal tissue following combination therapy with emphasis on the role of irradiation combined with chemotherapy. *Cancer* 37:1201–1213, 1976.

14 Radiation Therapy in Less Common Primary Bone Tumors

J. Robert Cassady, M.D.

1. Non-Hodgkin's lymphoma
   (reticulum cell sarcoma) of bone
2. Giant cell tumor of bone
3. Aneurysmal bone cyst
4. Histiocytosis X

A number of less common benign and malignant primary bone neoplasms may be seen on occasion in a busy tumor clinic. This chapter will assess the efficacy and role of irradiation in the treatment of the more frequently encountered of these conditions.

NON-HODGKIN'S LYMPHOMA OF BONE

Non-Hodgkin's lymphoma (reticulum cell sarcoma) of bone is less common than Ewing's sarcoma, but it shows many radiographic and, on occasion, histologic similarities to the latter. Significant differences appear to exist in natural history between the pediatric and the adult forms of this disease.[1] In the young, a significant incidence of leukemic conversion occurs, as with other non-Hodgkin's lymphomas of childhood. Most often a long bone is involved, and the femur is the most commmonly affected. Although the lesion is usually monostotic, a small but significant number of patients with multiple bone involvement are seen (Figure 1).[2] Ewing's sarcoma may also infrequently present with multiple tumors.

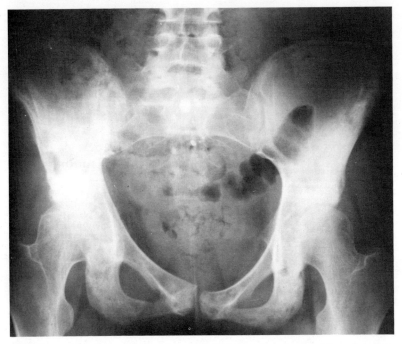

Figure 1. Multifocal involvement from non-Hódgkin's lymphoma of bone in pelvic bones of a teenage girl. The patient has been continuously free of disease for two years following radiation treatment. A dose of 5,000 rad was given to the entire pelvis in 25 fractions during a period of five weeks. Multiagent chemotherapy with Adriamycin, vincristine, and prednisone was also given.

Radiation therapy is widely recognized as the primary treatment of choice, as it produces local control and carries the obvious advantage of limb preservation.[1-3] Primary non-Hodgkin's lymphoma of bone usually arises in the medullary diaphyseal portions. Accordingly, the radiation portals, as in Ewing's sarcoma, should initially include the entire bone and necessary adjacent soft tissue, and care should be taken to preserve a strip of nonirradiated skin and subcutaneous tissue. However, lymph node spread is significantly more common with this disease, and it is our policy, when feasible, to irradiate the regional tier of lymph nodes of the affected bone during the period of initial treatment.[1,4] A radiotherapy dose of from 3,500 to 4,000 rad is administered during four to five weeks to this initial volume. The radiation field is then limited to the site of known tumor (with an appropriate margin) for an additional 1,500 to 2,000 rad over ten days. All of the technical details of irradiation of any primary bone tumor must also be observed in the treatment of this tumor (see Chapter 13). Local failure, seen in 5% to 20% of patients treated for Ewing's sarcoma, is rare in appropriately treated patients with non-Hodgkin's lymphoma of bone.

In the adult, relapse appears most often in another bone and/or in regional lymph nodes. In one series, 18 of 32 patients developed their first relapse in another bone, and one patient developed seven successive relapses in several different bones.[2] In the child, the development of multiple sites of failure, including leukemic conversion, is more common.[5] Consequently, it is our policy to treat such patients with chemotherapeutic regimens similar to those utilized for the treatment of leukemia or lymphoma.[6] In most patients, this does *not* include "prophylactic" treatment of the central nervous system with cranial irradiation.

In published series of treated patients, 35% to 50% have survived five or more years following treatment.[1-3] Late relapse is not uncommon.[7] The disease is often unpredictable, and even patients with multiple sites of involvement can survive disease-free for many years if treated aggressively.[3] We have seen and treated nine children with primary non-Hodgkin's lymphoma of bone, two of whom presented with contiguous multiple bone lesions. All patients are currently living without disease, from six months to over six years following irradiation. No patient has developed local failure.

GIANT CELL TUMOR OF BONE

Considerable controversy surrounds the natural history and pathology of, and the appropriate therapy for, this puzzling tumor. The tumor is virtually not seen prior to the time of epiphyseal closure, and females constitute the great majority of patients under age 20. Patients most commonly present in the third or early fourth decade.[8] The giant cell reparative granuloma (or giant cell epulis), affecting the mandible or maxilla, should be distinguished from this tumor, as it almost certainly represents a different entity. The "brown tumor" of hyperparathyroidism should also be excluded.

At presentation, 10% to 30% of these lesions will be regarded as frankly malignant.[8 9] However, metastases from multiple recurrent "benign" lesions after curettage are also recognized. In addition, apparently benign lesions have developed metastases following surgical therapy alone.[10 11] In fact, some pathologists feel that all giant cell lesions should be regarded as having malignant potential.*

Although complete excision or curettage of the primary lesion can be performed in the great majority of patients, local recurrence rates of 25% to 75% are commonly reported.[8 9 12 13] A wide range in the recurrence rate following irradiation has also been noted.[8 12 14 15]

---

*W. Meissner 1977: personal communication.

Interpretation of radiation therapy reports has been hampered by the early practice of delivering relatively small doses of radiation over a prolonged period (months to years). This treatment was accompanied by limited skin tolerance of the energy of orthovoltage equipment.

Malignant transformation following irradiation has also served to confuse the role of radiation therapy in the treatment of giant cell tumors. In light of current knowledge, it seems probable that historical reports of malignancy following irradiation represent an amalgam of true radiation-induced tumors, initially malignant lesions such as fibrosarcoma or osteosarcoma incorrectly interpreted as benign giant cell tumors, and true giant cell lesions which, in fact, were initially malignant but were interpreted pathologically as benign. Often there was only a short period between the irradiation of the primary lesion and the first evidence of malignant activity (usually development of metastatic disease) in many supposed radiation-transformed giant cell tumors. Most likely these lesions were malignant from the start and were wrongly interpreted histologically as benign, since true radiation-induced malignant lesions invariably require at least four and a half to five years to develop. It also appears possible that the techniques then employed for irradiation—the use of orthovoltage equipment with preferential bone absorption, as well as the practice of administering small doses of radiation over a long period—maximized the neoplastic potential of radiation therapy.

It is our current practice to recommend surgery (excision is preferred to curettage) in the initial management of extremity lesions where this is possible. Radiation therapy is reserved for cases where functional disability would be great following adequate surgery. Radiation therapy is also recommended for patients who have local recurrence despite apparently adequate surgery initially, or for those in whom complete tumor removal has not been possible. Finally, primary radiation therapy is advocated for surgically inaccessible or poorly accessible sites such as the spine or sacrum, or for large pelvic lesions.

Where radiation therapy is utilized, only megavoltage equipment is acceptable. The recommended dose is 4,500 to 5,500 rad given over five to six weeks. Radiation fields should encompass the entire bone lesion and any soft tissue extension. Rotational and other multifield radiation techniques should be used where possible to minimize adverse effects on normal tissue. The arc-wedge technique, for example, has many technical advantages in the treatment of spinal lesions.[16]

Several authors have noted the paradoxical radiographic increase in apparent tumor extent during radiation therapy.[15] [17] [18] This phenomenon is also commonly seen with Ewing's sarcoma, non-Hodgkin's lymphoma of bone, and other invasive lesions. It should not be construed as representing "resistance" or recurrence (extension) of tumor in response to irradiation. This misinterpretation has occasionally led to inappropriate surgery. When observed over a period of weeks to months, the "extension" almost invariably shows ultimate healing (Figure 2).

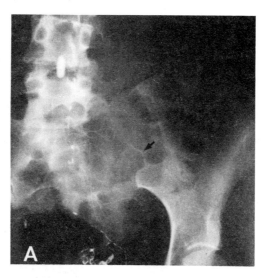

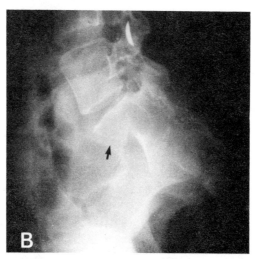

Figure 2. (A and B) Extensive giant cell tumor of bone centered in sacrum in a teenage girl (radiopaque suture material is visible in the center). Because of its location and size, primary radiation therapy was used to treat the lesion following biospy.

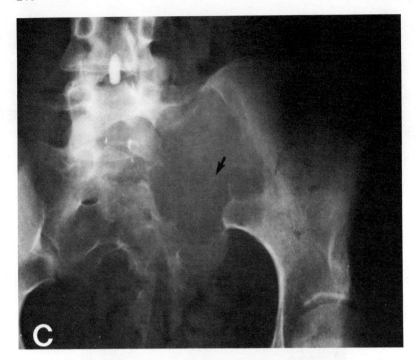

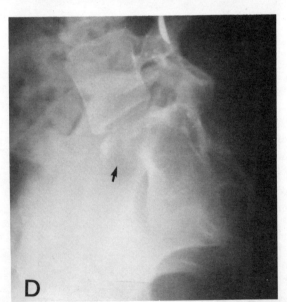

Figure 2 (C and D) Close to completion of the planned course (5,000 rad in 25 fractions during 5 weeks), radiographs demonstrate apparent increase in the size of the lesion and in the degree of bone destruction. Note disappearance of trabecular markings (arrow).

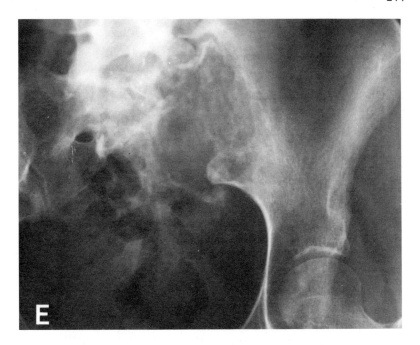

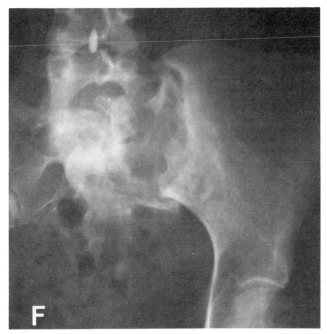

Figure 2 (E) Several weeks after completion of radiation therapy, there is clear evidence of healing of the lesion. **(F)** Radiographic appearance has been stable and the patient asymptomatic for several years.

ANEURYSMAL BONE CYST

This tumor possesses radiographic characteristics similar to those of giant cell tumor. However, it tends to affect a younger age group than that with giant cell tumor.[19] Spinal lesions are somewhat more common than others, and radiation therapy appears to have a primary role both for lesions in this site and for recurrent tumors. A radiation dose of from 2,500 to 3,000 rad given over a period of 18 to 24 days appears adequate in most patients.[19]

HISTIOCYTOSIS X

This unusual disease resembles both infection and tumor, and can be confused clinically and radiographically with a malignant bone tumor. Several forms of this condition present indications for radiation therapy.

Solitary eosinophilic granuloma of bone is usually seen in children older than 5 years of age. Radiation therapy is recommended in the following cases: if the lesion appears in a surgically inaccessible site; if it recurs following surgery; or if it poses a threat of pathologic fracture. Similarly, in the younger child with Hand-Schüller-Christian syndrome, radiation treatment of a long bone, a vertebra, the mastoid, or a soft tissue mass may be necessary. Irradiation of the hypothalamic and pituitary area may cause reversal of diabetes insipidus related to histiocytosis X if treatment is instituted soon after the onset of symptoms. Similarly, treatment of disease in the gums (and mandible or maxilla) may prevent loss of teeth and avoid major dental problems.

Although some authors recommend higher doses, 600 to 900 rad to the affected site appears adequate.[20-22] Local recurrences have been noted following 450 rad, but we have seen only rare local recurrences following 600 rad and we know of no local failure following delivery of 900 rad during a period of three to six days.[23] For this reason we recommend this dose for potentially critical areas such as the orbit or spine. A dose of 600 rad given in three fractions appears sufficient for most other sites. Megavoltage equipment is used for all patients.

REFERENCES

1. Wang, C.C. and Fletcher, D.J.: Primary reticulum cell sarcoma of bone. *Cancer* 22:994–998, 1968.

2. Newall, J., Friedman, M., and Navaez, F.: Extra-lymph-node reticulum cell sarcoma. *Radiology* 91:708–712, 1968.

3. Boston, H.C., Dahlin, D.C., Ivins, J.C. et al: Malignant lymphoma (so-called reticulum cell sarcoma) of bone. *Cancer* 34:1131–1137, 1974.

4. McCormack, L.J., Ivins, J.C., Kahlin, D. et al: Primary reticulum cell sarcoma of bone. *Cancer* 5:1182–1192, 1952.

5. Wollner, N., Burchenal, J., Leiberman, P.H. et al: Non-Hodgkin's lymphoma in children. *Med Pediatr Oncol* 1:235–263, 1975.

6. Jaffe, N., Buell, D., Cassady, J.R. et al: The role of staging in non-Hodgkin's lymphoma of childhood. *Cancer Treat Rep* 61:1001–1007, 1977.

7. Newall, J. and Friedman, M.: Reticulum cell sarcoma. *Radiology* 97:99–102, 1970.

8. Hutter, R.V.P., Worcester, J., Francis, K. et al: Benign and malignant giant cell tumor of bone. *Cancer* 15:653–690, 1962.

9. Larsson, S.E., Lorentzon, R., Boquist, L. et al: Giant cell tumor of bone. *J Bone Joint Surg* 57A:167–172, 1975.

10. Gresan, A.A., Dahlin, D.C., Lowell, F.A.P. et al: Benign giant cell tumor of bone metastasizing to lung. *Ann Thorac Surg* 16:531–535, 1973.

11. Kutchemesugi, A.D., Wright, J.R., Humphrey, R.L. et al: Pulmonary metastases from a well-differentiated giant cell tumor of bone. Report of a patient with apparent response to cyclophosphamide therapy. *Johns Hopkins Med J* 134:237–245, 1974.

12. Goldenberg, R.R., Campbell, C.J., Bonfiglio, M. et al: Giant cell tumor of bone. *J Bone Joint Surg* 52A:619–664, 1970.

13. Dahlin, D.C., Cupps, R.E., Johnson, E.W., Jr. et al: Giant cell tumor: a study of 195 cases. *Cancer* 25:1061–1070, 1970.

14. Friedman, M. and Pearlman, A.W.: Benign giant cell tumor of bone: radiation dose for each type. *Radiology* 91:1151–1158, 1968.

15. Buschke, F. and Cantril, S.T.: Roentgentherapy of benign giant cell tumor of bone. *Cancer* 2:293–315, 1949.

16. Larsen, R.D., Svensson, G.K., and Bjarngard, B.: The use of wedge filters to improve dose distribution with the partial rotation technique. *Radiology* 117:441–445, 1975.

17. Ellis, F.: Treatment of osteoclastoma by irradiation. *J Bone Joint Surg* 31B:268–280, 1949.

18. Morton, J.J.: Giant cell tumor of bone. *Cancer* 9:1012–1026, 1956.

19. Nobler, M.P., Higginbotham, N.L., and Phillips, R.F.: The cure of aneurysmal bone cyst. *Radiology* 90:1185–1192, 1968.

20. McGavatan, M.H. and Spady, H.A.: Eosinophilic granuloma

of bone: a study of 28 cases. *J Bone Joint Surg* 42A: 979–992, 1960.

21. Arcomano, J.P., Barnett, J.C., and Wunderlich, H.O.: Histiocytosis X. *Am J Roentgenol* 85:663–679, 1961.

22. Jones, J.C., Lilly, G.E., and Marlette, R.H.: Histiocytosis X. *J Oral Surg* 28:461–469, 1970.

23. Smith, D.G., Nesbit, M., D'Angio, G.J. et al: Histiocytosis X: role of radiation therapy in management with special reference to dose levels employed. *Radiology* 106:419–422, 1973.

15 Immunotherapy in Osteosarcoma

John G. Camblin, M.D.
and William F. Enneking, M.D.

1. Nonspecific agents
2. Tumor vaccination
   a. Intact cells
   b. Subcellular components
   c. Oncolysates
3. Serotherapy
4. Interferon therapy
5. Leukophoresis
6. Transfer factor

Nature has provided, in the white corpuscles as you call
them—in the phagocytes as we call them—a natural
means of devouring and destroying all diseased germs.
There is at bottom only one genuinely scientific treatment
for all diseases, and this is to stimulate the phagocytes.

George Bernard Shaw
The Doctor's Dilemma

The five-year survival rate of patients with osteosarcoma has
changed relatively little since the beginning of the century, when it
was about 5%.[1] Many series now record only a 10% to 20% five-
year survival rate, despite modern techniques encompassing
radiotherapy, surgery, and chemotherapy.[2] The predicted figure for
success of modern multidrug chemotherapy at five years was initially set about 80%, but unfortunately the results of trials followed
for at least three years have now shown that this estimate was
overoptimistic. In light of the apparent limitations of current

therapeutic regimens, then, one is prompted to "stimulate the phagocytes," or in modern terminology, to employ immunologic measures. This chapter will review the current methods by which the immune system may be stimulated and will report on the effectiveness of the different modalities.

NONSPECIFIC AGENTS

Numerous nonspecific agents, including transfer factor and interferon, have been investigated in the treatment of osteosarcoma. One of the earliest agents used was Coley's toxin, an extract of staphylococci.[3] This allegedly gave the immune system a general boost by presenting a direct antigenic challenge to the lymphocytes, and once activated, these immune cells would have an increased activity against tumor cell antigens. In the early 1900s the toxins were used against a wide variety of tumors with varying results. The results however, were not impressive enough to stimulate further research in this direction.

Nowell was the first to use the extract of the red kidney bean, *Phaseolus vulgaris,* to stimulate lymphocytes; since then, other plant alkaloids have also been employed for this purpose.[4] The extract initially used, phytohemagglutinin, was soon followed by concanavallin A, pokeweed mitogen, *Corynebacterium paruulum,* and others. They have been used with partial success in vivo and in vitro to stimulate lymphocyte activity against tumor cell lines. However, the medium in culture vessels is limited, and the products of metabolic activity of the stimulated cells, plus their use of the nutrients within the medium, may also direct cytotoxic activity against other competitive cells. Phytohemagglutinin will still stimulate nonsensitized cells to a degree of cytotoxicity against tumor cells in vitro, as will thymosin solution obtained from homogenized bovine thymus tissue.[5]

The major nonspecific immunotherapeutic agent at this time is undoubtedly bacillus Calmette-Guérin (BCG). Retrospective studies in the past few years have suggested that children who have been immunized with BCG against tuberculosis have had a lower than average incidence of leukemia.[6-8] Undoubtedly, as is the case with many retrospective studies, the comparison controls were not matched, and prospective data are still unavailable for analysis at this time. Nonetheless, BCG has found favor with a great many tumor research centers, partly because of its availability and general safety. It has been used as an adjunct to therapy for a wide range of tumors. At a recent cancer symposium where reports on 30 studies on tumor immunology were presented, BCG was reported to have been included as part of the protocol in all but 2 studies. All had a universal lack of success.[9]

It is widely recognized that injection of BCG directly into a skin nodule causes a local inflammatory reaction and results in nodule regression.[7] It does not alter the status of any other tumor nodules or metastases that may be present. A recent study which combined BCG with multidrug chemotherapy reports a 17% partial remission rate.[10] Sparks et al and others have used skin sensitization as the mode of administration of BCG, but photographs of the resulting skin lesions would indicate that the "cure" this produces is about as bad as the disease.[11]

Osteosarcoma has not escaped the enthusiasm for BCG as a therapy. All authors report increased cell-mediated immunity after such therapy, especially in patients tested with purified protein derivative. These patients also have been shown to respond to other skin-testing agents, such as dinitrochlorobenzene (DNCB).[12][13] When used in conjunction with a tumor cell vaccine, BCG has been reported to increase survival time.[14][15] In all studies so far, however, the numbers of subjects have been small and the follow-up periods short, therefore the results cannot yet be statistically analyzed.

One criticism of BCG therapy and sensitivity testing is that the patient responses have not necessarily correlated with antitumor activity. In fact, Stewart and colleagues have demonstrated that many tumor patients can show reactivity to BCG, be immunized to BCG, and be sensitized to DNCB until terminal stages of the disease.[16][17] These authors have demonstrated also that these same patients had varied responses to skin tests with tumor antigen solution and that activity to the antigen was associated with the patient's well-being. Thus, tumor antigen sensitivity was lost long before the patients reached advanced stages of illness and long before they lost reactivity to standard skin-testing agents such as DNCB and BCG. Many other agents, including C. paruulum, have been tried for antitumor activity without success and are still under investigation.

BCG is used in a wide variety of dosages, regimens, and modes of administration. The latter range from direct intratumor injection, to skin scarification, to inhalation. There are several sources of BCG, all manufactured in varying degrees of concentration and purity. These facts cast some doubt on BCG's efficacy as an immuno-therapeutic agent. It would appear that to achieve a standard of comparison with other BCG studies, in addition to stipulating the exact concentration of BCG used and the mode and frequency of administration, one should specify also the source of manufacture. If the work of Stewart and associates is confirmed, and antitumor recognition and BCG recognition are not synonymous, then this therapeutic agent, as has Coley's toxin, will fall into disuse.[16]

TUMOR VACCINATION

Intact Cells

Information is available to suggest that tumor-specific and tumor-associated antigens and antibodies are present in a tumor-bearing host. Eilber and Morton have found that antibodies to osteosarcoma were present in all of the osteosarcoma patients they tested and in 85% of normal, healthy family members.[18] In contrast, antibody was present in only 29% of normal blood donors. Similar results have been reported by Friedman and Carter, who found that 92% of patients with osteosarcoma reacted to the tumor by antibody production.[12] Antibodies were detected in 21% of normal blood donors in their study. Titers recorded were up to 1:256 for patients and 1:128 for family members, as compared with a mean value of only 1:19 for normal subjects.

It follows logically from the concept of sensitization that one should be able to subject a patient to challenge with a specific tumor antigen and thus render the patient immune to the particular tumor type. This concept is not new; it was originally conceived at the beginning of the century, even though there was no real understanding of the immune system at that time. More recently, however, the concept of immunization against tumor has been revised. A study has been reported of 12 patients who were vaccinated intradermally with whole, irradiated human melanoma or osteosarcoma cells that had been harvested from tissue culture.[19] The radiation dose was 5,000 rad and the osteosarcoma cells were then given to 5 osteosarcoma patients and the melanoma cells to 7 melanoma patients. Following a treatment period of 5 to 7 months, all the patients developed a delayed hypersensitivity reaction at the metastatic sites of their respective tumors. Two patients with osteosarcoma remained without evidence of disease for 18 months, and without further lesion development for two years. The disease progressed in the other patients and they eventually died.[19]

Immunoprophylactic administration of intact tumor cells before there is tumor challenge has been shown to be effective in the laboratory.[20][21] It also has been effective even when given several days after a tumor challenge.[22] A study carried out in 29 osteosarcoma patients with metastatic disease used both BCG and cultured human osteosarcoma cells as immunizing agents.[23] Although there was some suggestion of a prolonged disease-free period—8.1 months, 3.1 without immunotherapy—the difference was not statistically significant. Many pitfalls threaten this type of protocol, including the variable amount of tumor present (even in those patients classified as disease-free) and also the exact mode and frequency of delivery of the immunizing agent.

Subcellular Components

A variety of experiments have shown that animals can be successfully immunized against tumors with cell homogenates or membrane fraction as well as with whole, killed tumor cells; yet it has not been possible to do this in man. Possible reasons for this failure include variations in tumor cell antigenicity and in the amount of tumor in each patient at the time they were treated. Also, humans are not genetically identical, as are the majority of experimental animals in the series used in the various reported investigations.

Oncolysates

Investigators have attempted to make the tumor cell more strongly antigenic, using BCG, other nonspecific stimulants, and viral oncolysates.[14][24] Results of the use of influenza virus in animal experiments have been encouraging.[25] Within the experimental setting, viral oncolysate injection protected mice from cancer challenge, and when the surviving animals were rechallenged, they were again found to be immune. Viruses obtained from the oncolysate and given to the tumor cells have also yielded protection against tumor challenge.[24] Similar results have been noted with use of bovine enterovirus. It is thought that the growing virus budding on the surface of the tumor cell in some way modifies or accentuates the tumor-specific antigens by acting as a hapten or by unmasking or removing factors inhibiting the antigenic capacity of the cells.

Viral oncolysate therapy has been tried in osteosarcoma patients. No evidence of toxicity has been found, and 5 of 12 patients developed antisarcoma antibody and cellular immunity to their tumor.[24] The survival figures are not as yet statistically significant. When type A influenza virus was used in conjunction with BCG and chemotherapy, those treated with the oncolysates did slightly better than those in the control regimens, but this difference also is not as yet statistically significant.[14]

Over the years many attempts have been made to produce a vaccine for use against tumors. Tumor vaccination has been shown to be effective in the laboratory setting, but not in clinical circumstances. It does not appear to show any more promise than serum therapy or the use of nonspecific immunostimulating agents such as BCG and concanavallin A. It still remains to be seen how tumor vaccination will compare to transfer factor, immune RNA transfer, and other modes of adoptive therapy.

SEROTHERAPY

Serotherapy was first attempted around 1895, without any success, using dog and goat serum from immunized animals. Since that time, little progress has been made in this direction, in spite of numerous efforts. It has been shown repeatedly that antibody is produced against both animal and human tumors, including osteosarcoma.[23] [26] This antibody is cytotoxic in vitro, but thus far there is no real evidence of any effectiveness in vivo. A few reports suggest that it may be beneficial in some leukemias and in melanoma, where metastases may regress or disappear after antibody production and subsequent removal of the primary lesion.[27]

In a trial at the University of Florida, a series of 18 patients with osteosarcoma was treated initially with conventional surgery (usually amputation or hip disarticulation, depending on the site of the lower limb lesion) and then with serotherapy.* In all cases the patients were under 21 years of age and had a clear chest x-ray film and a solitary primary tumor diagnosed histologically as an osteosarcoma. These patients were given infusions (three doses at weekly intervals) of 500 ml of plasma obtained from disease-free relatives or normal blood donors. Some of the plasma was shown by passive hemagglutination assay to contain antibodies to osteosarcoma antigen, and the control serum was shown not to contain such antibody. At the end of one year no difference could be demonstrated between the test and the control groups. However, no patient's condition was worsened, and only one had a slight reaction to the infused plasma. This project, like others before it, was abandoned.

INTERFERON THERAPY

"Interferon" is the name given to a soluble, heat-labile fraction (or fractions) created by the reaction between chicken chorioallantoic tissue and inactivated influenza virus.[28] [29] It is so called because it in some way interferes with the ability of the virus to penetrate and infect cells. It first came to the attention of investigators because of its ability to block the multiplication of influenza and related myxoviruses. Interferons are species-specific but will react against many types of viruses within the species from which they are prepared. It is

---

*J.G. Camblin and W.F. Enneking 1976: unpublished data.

believed that in vitro cell cultures and host tissue cells produce interferons in response to exposure to a viral agent, whether the agent is an infecting one or not.[28]

Initially interferon was produced by incubating a stimulating virus (such as influenza) with tissue culture cells and extracting the crude reaction product from the supernatant fluid after a suitable period.[28] [29] More recently, interferon has been successfully produced in usable quantities from human leukocytes.[30] [31] It also may be produced from a wide variety of other cell types.[31]

The exact nature of interferon is not known, but research has shown it to be a protein: it is not denatured by antiviral antibodies; it does not form precipitate in the presence of viral particles; and it is not self-replicating. Interferon is nondialyzable, it is destroyed by proteolytic enzymes such as trypsin, and it is inactivated when heated to 60 C for one hour.[28] [30] [32] Cells treated with interferon are known to be resistant to infection with related viruses. It is thought that viral antigen may promote a signal in the untreated cells that activates chromosome 5 to produce messenger RNA, which migrates to the ribosomes and directs them to produce interferon (Figure 1). The interferons so produced then activate other non-invaded cells at the site of chromosome 21 to cause synthesis of an antiviral protein.[30] [31]

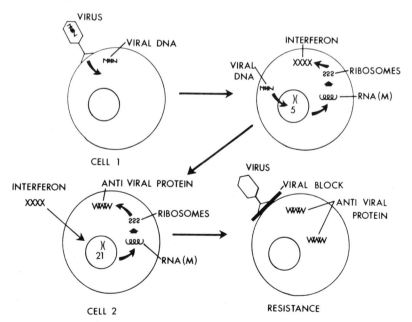

Figure 1 Schematic diagram of interferon production and mechanism of action.

Human interferon, the international standard prepared from leukocytes, is fully active in man and is only slightly so in other higher primates.[33] Animal experiments have shown that interferon can have some antitumor activity.[33-35] Many tumors in animals have been ascribed to viral agents, but in spite of considerable research in this direction, there is only limited proof that this is the case in man.

Strander and colleagues have conducted a noncontrolled clinical trial in 11 patients with osteosarcoma.[36] The patients received intramuscular doses of 2.5×10^6 IU of human interferon prepared from leukocytes on three occasions per week over a period of 18 months. Seven of these patients were disease-free at the end of that time. In another study, these same investigators have attempted to reduce the rate of infection in patients with osteosarcoma by means of interferon therapy, and they have used members of the patients' families in the same household as controls.[37] The patients have been treated for up to two years, and the results so far suggest that they have benefited from this treatment, as they have had fewer infections then have the untreated controls. No patient in either of these studies has had any adverse reaction to the interferon itself. However, the authors acknowledge that the numbers of subjects in the studies are few and that the nature of the symptoms under investigation is not specific. Further data on clinical trials such as these may be forthcoming, though, since human interferon can now be obtained commercially.

LEUKOPHORESIS

In addition to the studies on active immunization, several lines of research have developed on passive transfer of tumor immunity by whole blood or blood products. One of the earliest of these studies was carried out in Scotland by Woodruff and Nolan, who used white-cell suspensions obtained from the spleens of immunocompetent patients and transfused these into other patients of similar ABO blood groups.[38] It was hoped that the cells from the immunocompetent patients would boost immune capability in the recipients. It did not, for a variety of reasons. One was that the study involved only patients with widespread disease, and the ratio of active cells transfused to tumor mass was low. In addition, this therapy was administered in conjunction with steroids or cytotoxic drugs, both of which are lymphocytotoxic.

Repeatedly, studies involving transfused leukocytes have shown transfer of skin sensitivities with only temporary or minimal antitumor activity, probably because of dilution of the transfused cells with nonlymphoid cells and also nonreactive or uncommitted lymphoid cells, which cannot act against a tumor.[27] [39] [40] [41] Investigators postulate that a ratio of lymphocytes to tumor cells of at least 25:1 should be achieved. In general, lymphocyte transfusion for osteosarcoma has not had significant success, although some good results have been recorded.[42] Leukocytes obtained from a long-time osteosarcoma survivor were transfused into his brother, who had developed osteosarcoma; the brother had been in complete remission for two years when the follow-up report was made. Experimentally, tumor growth has been delayed but not halted by the transfusion of active whole leukocytes or the products of lysed cells.[43] [44]

A study was instituted at the University of Florida in 1969 with 32 osteosarcoma patients.[45] These patients were surgically treated according to standard therapy, and each received tumor implants from another patient. Lymphocytes or leukocytes were obtained from those who were sensitized to the implants, and the leukocyte-rich plasma was then infused into the original tumor tissue donor. Skin tests showed a transfer of PPD, coccidioidin, and histoplasmin sensitivity. The patients were also skin-tested with tumor antigens before and after lymphocyte transfer. The skin test results showed only variable transfer of sensitivity to the skin test antigens, which included tumor antigen extract to which three patients had a positive response.

Comparisons at five years showed no statistical differences in initial results between the test group and historical controls. However, the test group was shown to be marginally benefited by this mode of treatment when results from later phases of the study were compared. This test group consisted of both patients who had metastatic disease at diagnosis and others who developed metastatic sites within the first three months after diagnosis. When the remaining 28 patients without metastatic spread initially were compared with 28 age- and sex-matched controls from other centers, four-year disease-free rates of 44% vs 10% were observed (Figure 2). The mean time until metastasis was 6 ± 2 months in the case of historical controls and 15 ± 2 months in the case of those receiving immunotherapy.

The question that arises is: why has this group benefited more than others treated by similar measures? One possibility is, of course, that of sample variation, and if the study had been carried out with a large number of patients, the results might have been different. Other reasons may be that (1) most of the patients in this study were under 21 years of age, (2) the site of the osteosarcoma was in a single long bone, and (3) chest x-ray films were clear at the time of diagnosis. Another factor of interest is that this particular

224

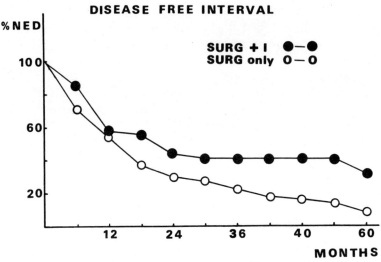

Figure 2 Comparison of osteosarcoma patients treated by surgery and leukophoresis at the University of Florida with age- and sex-matched patients treated by surgery alone.

study group received tumor implants not in a single site but in multiple fragments. Follow-up with assessment of immunologic factors is still being carried out in this particular patient group.[45]

TRANSFER FACTOR

Transfer factor has been described by Lawrence, who found that lymphocyte activity to an antigen challenge could be transferred to a nonsensitized lymphoid cell by using a dialyzable extract of sensitized lymphoid cells.[46] Thus the nonreactive subject could be made reactive. Little additional progress was made until recently because of the difficulty in isolating purified fractions of the crude extracts.[47] We still lack data on the exact identity of transfer factor, its mode of action, and its optimal dosage and mode of administration.

Many factors have been reported as being released from sensitized lymphoid T cells. Among these are skin permeability factors which facilitate access to affected areas, and macrophage control factors which both stimulate macrophage and polymorphonuclear cells to invade damaged tissue and also retain them there. Other substances released include osteoclast activity factor, collagen-synthesizing factor, interferon, and transfer factor.[48] Unfortunately, the identification and characterization of these substances have proved difficult.

Transfer factor is a low molecular weight (10,000 to 12,000), dialyzable product released when peripheral blood leukocytes are lysed.[49][50] It is prepared by collecting the buffy coat from whole blood by the Ficoll-Hypaque method, or by using continuous cell separators and then lysing the cells by successive freezing and thawing.[50-53] Finally, the free fluid is dialyzed against normal saline, and the resulting supernatant liquid containing the lysed cell products is used as transfer factor. The exact nature and method of operation of this transfer is not known, and thus far at least 20 different types have been reported.[54] One of the difficulties in collecting purified transfer factor is that the buffy coat, although constituted of 95% lymphocytes, is contaminated by other leukocyte cell types containing a wide variety of enzymes. Therefore, the end product transfer factor may not be identical to that which was originally present in the sensitized T cells.

Interest in transfer factor was revived in 1970 when it was used to treat the Wiskott-Aldrich syndrome, a sex-linked immune deficiency disease.[17][48] Since then many authors have reported its use in transfer, from reactive donors to nonreactive subjects, of specific sensitivities to a wide range of antigens.[55] It has also been reported that transfer factor may be nonspecific regarding antigen transfer and that the resulting sensitivity may derive from recipient cell activity as well as donor recognition.[56] In addition to its assessment in a wide range of infectious diseases, transfer factor has been applied to the treatment of cancer in general and to that of osteosarcoma in particular.

One of the earliest assessments or transfer factor in osteosarcoma was carried out in 1976 by Fudenberg, who suggested a possible viral etiology for this disease.[48] Transfer factor donors were selected on the basis of their cytotoxic reaction to osteosarcoma cells. In the natural state of the disease, osteosarcoma patients initially were cytotoxic to their cell line (and 25% of their household contacts also demonstrated a cytotoxic response to osteosarcoma cells), but over a period of time this reactivity was lost. This loss of reactivity was usually detected shortly before onset of metastatic disease. When transfer factor was used, cytotoxic sensitivity could be transferred from the reactive donors to the osteosarcoma patient and thus prolong their period of cytotoxic reactivity against osteosarcoma. However, the ultimate prognosis and outcome in these patients have not yet been reported.

More recently, transfer factor has been evaluated in a wide variety of malignancies, including melanoma, osteosarcoma, and several types of carcinoma.[53] Thirteen patients responded with a 25% to 75% reduction of tumor mass during the period of treatment. The remainder, most of whom showed blocking on lymphocyte proliferative response testing, did not respond. Five patients experienced either total regression or a stasis of metastatic growth for up to eight months. The suggestion from this study is that subcutaneous injections of transfer factor at two-week intervals may be a useful therapeutic approach after removal of the primary lesion, and before metastases have become established.

Levin and co-workers have reported enhanced cellular immunity to osteosarcoma when transfer factor from patients' relatives was administered.[57] Further, biopsy samples revealed that this mode of treatment induced lymphocyte infiltration into osteosarcoma tissue, although this in itself does not guarantee that these cells were engaged in antitumor activity.[58][59] The patients were followed up for two years. Of the 11 in the study, 4 patients in whom transfer factor alone was used are still tumor-free, and 2 others are without evidence of disease after surgical resection of pulmonary metastases.

While it is too early to determine the true value of transfer factor in osteosarcoma therapy, it does appear to show promise.[60] All authors are in agreement as to its safety—no reactions to the dialyzable extract have been reported so far.[49] Alteration of the recipient's immune response has been shown to be induced by transfer factor, and partial control of disease has been recorded. Transfer factor may thus be a potentially useful tool, but more work is required in this area to determine its nature, its mode of action, and optimal dosage and mode of administration. Additional and carefully controlled clinical trials with transfer factor are required to establish a true basis for comparison with current chemotherapeutic regimens. Follow-up of at least two years will be needed in all cases, and the studies should include larger numbers of patients than have so far been reported.[60][61]

CONCLUSION

We have set out to review the history and the various modalities of immunotherapy. Immunotherapy, even when the same reactive agents have been used, has varied considerably. Clearly, the host does mount an immune reaction, both by cellular immunity and by antibody production to the tumor that is present, but unfortunately this does not appear to be able to successfully deal with overt neoplasia. In fact, there are numerous references to augmentation of tumor by antibody, which although present in varying quantities, apparently does not kill the tumor cells but instead serves to protect them from direct cellular immunity, which appears to be slightly more effective than antibody in achieving tumor cell death.[62-64]

Of the various modes of immunotherapy, passive immunotherapy using serum appears to be, at most, only a short-lived process, and so far has not proved effective. More encouraging results are being produced with adoptive immunotherapy in the form of either interferon, leukophoresis, or transfer factor, all of which are still in the early stages of investigation. The various antibody studies do indicate that the cause of osteosarcoma in man may be viral in part. This conclusion is based on the reactivity shown not only by the patient but also by their disease-free family members within the same household. Should such a virus ever be discovered, it should, theoretically, be possible to produce a vaccine against it and thus produce immunity to this form of tumor. It is more likely, however, that in the immediate future antibody or immune detection will be used more for diagnosis or for monitoring progression of the disease.

The concept of immunochemotherapy remains largely uninvestigated. In theory, chemotherapeutic agents could be attached to antibody of a particular tumor and the antibody could then carry the chemotherapeutic agent directly to the tumor cell, where it would bring about tumor cell death rather than the immune reaction of the antibody itself. Considerable work remains to be done in all of these directions before solution to this problem is achieved.

REFERENCES

1. Duthie, R.B. and Ferguson, A.B.: *Orthopaedic Surgery*. 7th ed. Edward Arnold, London, 1973, pp 594–618.

2. Sweetnam, R.D.: Tumors of bone and their management. *Ann R Coll Surg Engl* 54:63–71, 1974.

3. Nauts, H.C.: Beneficial effects of immunotherapy (bacterial toxins) in sarcoma of soft tissues other than lymphosarcoma. *Natl Cancer Inst Monogr* vol. 16, 1975.

4. Nowell, P.C.:Phytohemagglutinin: an indicator of mitosis in cultures of normal lymphocytes. *Cancer Res* 20:462–466, 1960.

5. Camblin, J.G.: Immunological Aspects of Osteosarcoma. Ph.D. dissertation, Queen's University of Belfast, 1975.

6. Davignon, L., Lemonde, P., Robilland, P. et al: BCG vaccination and leukemia mortality. *Lancet* 2:638, 1970.

7. McKhann, C.F. and Gunnarsson, A.: Approaches to immunotherapy. *Cancer* 34:1521–1531, 1974.

8. Rosenthal, S.R.: BCG vaccine. *Am Fam Physician* 5:98–103, 1972.

9. Proceedings of the Illinois Cancer Symposium, 1977. In Crispen, R.G. (ed): *Neoplasm Immunity: Solid Tumor Therapy.* Franklin Institute Press, Philadelphia, 1977, pp 1–266.

10. Song, J. and Choi, C.: Immunochemotherapy in patients with advanced breast cancer. In Crispen, R.G. (ed: *Neoplasm Immunity: Solid Tumor Therapy.* Franklin Institute Press, Philadelphia, 1977, pp 161–167.

11. Sparks, F., Pardridge, D., Wile, A. et al: Immunotherapy of human breast cancer with BCG and viable and irradiated tumor cell vaccines. In Crispen, R.G. (ed): *Neoplasm Immunity: Solid Tumor Therapy.* Franklin Institute Press, Philadelphia, 1977, pp 179–188.

12. Friedman, M.A. and Carter, S.K.: The therapy of osteogenic sarcoma: current status and thoughts for the future. *J Surg Oncol* 4:482–510, 1972.

13. Sokal, J.E. and Aungst, C.W.: Immunotherapy with cultured human cells and BCG. *Transplant Proc* 7:317–321, 1975.

14. Sinkovics, J., Plager, C., and Romero, J.: Immunology and immunotherapy of patients with sarcomas. In Crispen, R.G. (ed): *Neoplasm Immunity: Solid Tumor Therapy.* Franklin Institute Press, Philadelphia, 1977, pp 211–219.

15. Townsend, C.M. and Eilber, F.R.: Adjuvant immunotherapy for skeletal sarcomas, abstract 1162. *Proc Am Assoc Cancer Res* 16:261, 1976.

16. Stewart, T.H.M., Hollinshead, A., Harris, J. et al: A survival study of specific active immunochemotherapy in lung cancer. In Crispen, R.G. (ed): *Neoplasm Immunity: Solid Tumor Therapy.* Franklin Institute Press, Philadelphia, 1977, pp 37–48.

17. Spitler, L.E., Levin, A.S., Stites, D.P. et al: The Wiskott-Aldrich syndrome: results of transfer factor therapy. *J Clin Invest* 51:3216–3224, 1972.

18. Eilber, F.R. and Morton, D.L.: Immunologic studies of human sarcomas: additional evidence suggesting an associated sarcoma virus. *Cancer* 26:588–596, 1970.

19. Gerner, R.E., Moore, G.E., and Tarbon, D.S.: Delayed hypersensitivity reaction at metastatic tumor sites. *Rocky Mt Med J* 72:17–20, 1975.

20. Bell, E.C.: A normal adult and fetal lung antigen present at different quantitative levels in different histologic types of human lung cancer. *Cancer* 37:703–706, 1976.

21. Holmes, F.C., Kahan, B.D., and Morton, D.L.: Soluble tumor-specific transplantation antigens from guinea pig sarcomas. *Cancer* 25:373–379, 1975.

22. Wepsic, H.T., Kronman, B.S., Zbar, B. et al: Immunotherapy of an intramuscular tumor in strain 2 guinea pigs. *J Natl Cancer Inst*

45:377–386, 1970.

23. Eilber, F.R. and Morton, D.L.: Osteosarcoma: results of treatment employing adjuvant immunotherapy. *Clin Orthop* 111:94–100, 1975.

24. Green, A.A., Pratt, C., Webster, R.G. et al: Immunotherapy of osteosarcoma patients with virus-modified tumor cells. *Ann NY Acad Sci* 277:396–411, 1976.

25. Lindermann, J. and Klein, P.A.: Immunological aspects of viral oncolysates. *Recent Results Cancer Res* 9:1–84, 1967.

26. Camblin, J., Enneking, W., Forbes, J. et al: Immunodiagnosis of osteosarcoma. In R.G. Crispen (ed): *Neoplasm Immunity: Solid Tumor Therapy.* Franklin Institute Press, Philadelphia, 1977, pp 201–209.

27. Smith, G.V., Morse, P.A., Deraps, G.D. et al: Immunotherapy of patients with cancer. *Surgery* 74:59–68, 1973.

28. Ho, M.: Interferons. *N Engl J Med* 266:1258–1264, 1962.

29. Isaacs, A. and Lindenman, J.: Virus interference. I. The interferon. *Proc R Soc Lond [Biol]* 147:258–267A, 268–273B, 1957.

30. Burke, D.C.: The status of interferon. *Sci Am* 236:42–50, 1977.

31. Mogensen, K.E. and Cantell, K.: Human leukocyte interferon: a role for disulphide bonds. *J Gen Virol* 22:95–103, 1974.

32. Fantes, K.H.: Purification and properties of human interferon. *Ann NY Acad Sci* 173:118–121, 1970.

33. Strander, H., Cantell, K., Carlstrom, G. et al: Clinical and laboratory investigations on man: systemic administration of potent interferon to man. *J Natl Cancer Inst* 51:733–742, 1973.

34. Gresser, I. and Bourali, C.: Antitumor effects of interferon preparations in mice. *J Natl Cancer Inst* 45:365–376, 1970.

35. Gresser, I.: Antitumor effects of interferon. *Adv Cancer Res* 16:97–140, 1972.

36. Strander, H., Cantell, K., Jakobsson, P. et al: Exogenous interferon therapy of osteogenic sarcoma. *Acta Orthop Scand* 45:958–959, 1974.

37. Strander, H., Cantell, K., Carlstrom, G. et al: Acute infections in interferon-treated patients with osteosarcoma: preliminary report of a comparative study. *J Infect Dis* 133A(suppl): 245–248, 1976.

38. Woodruff, M.F.A. and Nolan, B.: Treatment of advanced cancer by injection of allogeneic spleen cells. *Lancet* 2:426–429, 1963.

39. Roth, J.A., Holmes, E.C., Reisfield, R. et al: Isolation of a soluble tumor-associated antigen from human melanoma. *Cancer* 37:104–110, 1976.

40. Sutherland, C.M., Krementz, E.T., Hornung, M.D. et al: Transfer of in vitro cytotoxicity against osteosarcoma cells. *Surgery* 79:682-685, 1976.

41. Moore, G.E. and Gerner, R.E.: Cancer immunity— hypothesis and clinical trial of lymphocytotherapy for malignant disease. *Ann Surg* 172:733-739, 1970.

42. Nadler, S.H. and Moore, G.E.: Immunotherapy of malignant disease. *Arch Surg* 99:376-381, 1969.

43. Greco, R.S. and Storer, E.H.: The effect of intact and lysed leukocytes on murine tumor growth and host survival. *J Surg Oncol* 7:67-76, 1975.

44. Kopf, A.W.: Immunotherapy for human malignant melanoma. *South Med J* 68:495-503, 1975.

45. Marsh, B., Flynn, L., and Enneking, W.F.: Immunologic aspects of osteosarcoma and their application on therapy. *J Bone Joint Surg* 54A:1367-1390, 1972.

46. Lawrence, H.S.: Supplemental general discussion. In Ascher, M.S., Gottlieb, A.A., and Kirkpatrick, C.H. (eds): *Transfer Factor: Basic Properties and Clinical Application.* Academic Press, New York, 1976, p 516.

47. Shifrine, M., Thilsted, J., and Pappagianis, D.: Canine transfer factor. In Ascher, M.S., Gottlieb, A.A., and Kirkpatrick, C.H. (eds): *Transfer Factor: Basic Properties and Clinical Applications.* Academic Press, New York, 1976, pp 349-357.

48. Fudenberg, H.H.: Dialyzable transfer factor in the treatment of human osteosarcoma: an analytical review. *Ann NY Acad Sci* 277:545-556, 1976.

49. LoBuglio, A.F. and Neidhart, J.A.: A review of transfer factor immunotherapy in cancer. *Cancer* 34:1563-1570, 1974.

50. Potter, H., Rosenfeld, S., and Dressler, D.: Transfer factor. *Ann Intern Med* 81:838-847, 1974.

51. Bearden, J.D., Thord, D.E., and Coltman, C.A.: Adjunctive transfer factor in osteogenic sarcoma. I. Clinical implications of chemotherapy and immunotherapy. In Ascher, M.D., Gottlieb, A.A., and Kirkpatrick, C.H. (eds): *Transfer Factor: Basic Properties and Clinical Applications* Academic Press, New York, 1976. pp 553-561.

52. Thor, D.E., Coltman, C.A., Bearden, J.D. et al: Adjunctive transfer factor in osteosarcoma. II. Methodology and results of the immunological studies. In Ascher, M.S., Gottlieb, A.A., and Kirkpatrick, C.H. (eds): *Transfer Factor: Basic Properties and Clinical Applications.* Academic Press, New York, 1976, pp 563-569.

53. Vetto, M., Burger, D.R., Nolte, J.E. et al: Transfer factor immunotherapy in cancer. In Ascher, M.S., Gottlieb, A.A., and Kirkpatrick, C.H. (eds): *Transfer Factor: Basic Properties and Clinical*

Applications. Academic Press, New York, 1976, pp 523–530.

54. Semih, E.: On the nature of transfer factor. In Ascher, M.S., Gottlieb, A.A., and Kirkpatrick, C.H. (eds): *Transfer Factor: Basic Properties and Clinical Applications.* Adademic Press, New York, 1976, pp 687–690.

55. Ascher, M.S., Gottlieb, A.A., and Kirkpatrick, C.H. (eds): *Transfer Factor: Basic Properties and Clinical Applications.* Academic Press, New York, 1976.

56. Salaman, M.R.: Specificity of transfer factor on lymphocyte transformation. In Ascher, M.S., Gottlieb, A.A., and Kirkpatrick, C.H. (eds): *Transfer Factor: Basic Properties and Clinical Application.* Academic Press, New York, 1976, pp 13–19.

57. Levin, A.S., Byers, V.S., Fudenberg, H.H. et al: Transfer factor therapy in osteogenic sarcoma. *Trans Assoc Am Phys* 88:153–157, 1974.

58. Levin, A.S.: Transfer factor therapy: current status. *South Med J* 68:1465–1467, 1975.

59. Levin, A.S., Byers, V.S., Fudenberg, H.H. et al: Osteogenic sarcoma: immunologic parameters before and during immunotherapy with tumor-specific transfer factor. *J Clin Invest* 55:487–499, 1975.

60. Byers, V.S., Levin, A.S., LeCam, L. et al: Tumor-specific transfer factor therapy in osteogenic sarcoma: a two-year study. *Ann NY Acad Sci* 277:621–627, 1976.

61. Ivins, J.C., Ritts, R.E., Prichard, D. et al: Transfer factor versus combination chemotherapy: a preliminary report of a randomized postsurgical adjuvant treatment study in osteosarcoma. *Ann NY Acad Sci* 277:558–574, 1976.

62. Baldwin, R.W. and Robins, R.A.: Factors interfering with immunological rejection of tumors. *Br Med Bull* 32:118–123, 1976.

63. Stevenson, G.T. and Laurence, D.J.R.: Report of a workshop on the immune response to solid tumors in man. *Int J Cancer* 16:887–896, 1975.

64. Suciu-Foca, N., Buda, J., McManus, J. et al: Impaired responsiveness of lymphocytes and serum inhibitory factors in patients with cancer. *Cancer Res* 33:2373–2377, 1973.

16 Management of Benign Bone Tumors in Children

Franklin H. Sim, M.D., Ronald B. Irwin, M.D.,
and David C. Dahlin, M.D.

1. General principles
2. Tumors of chondrogenic origin
3. Tumors of osteogenic origin
4. Tumors of fibrogenic origin
5. Tumors of vascular origin
6. Tumors of unknown origin
7. Conditions simulating benign bone tumors

INTRODUCTION

Benign tumors of bone in children, like those in adults, may arise from several histologic types (Table 1): chondrogenic, osteogenic, and fibrogenic, as well as from the main components of normal bone; but they may also arise from vascular, neurogenic, or lipogenic elements, or they may even be of unknown origin.[1-4] Conditions that simulate bone tumors also must be considered because these conditions cause equal concern and difficulty, both in diagnosis and treatment.

The problem of osseous tumors of childhood is magnified because their presence or treatment may have a profound influence on the growth potential of the affected part, as well as a great effect on the psychologic well-being of the child or adolescent at this already sensitive time of his or her life.

234

Table 1
Benign Bone Tumors of Childhood

Histologic Type	Tumors
Chondrogenic	Osteochondroma
	Chondroma
	Chondroblastoma
	Chondromyxoid fibroma
Osteogenic	Osteoid osteoma
	Osteoblastoma
Fibrogenic	Fibroma
	Desmoplastic fibroma
Vascular	Hemangioma
	Angioglomoid tumor (?)
Lymphatic	Lymphangioma
Lipogenic	Lipoma
Neurogenic	Neurilemoma
Unknown origin	Benign giant cell tumors
Conditions simulating primary bone tumors	Fibrous dysplasia
	Aneurysmal bone cysts
	Unicameral bone cysts
	Histiocytosis X

GENERAL PRINCIPLES

After the osseous lesion has been found, management demands evaluation clinically, roentgenographically, and pathologically, and treatment is based on an accurate histologic diagnosis of an adequate biopsy specimen. Bone tumors of children present a problem that is not greatly different from that in adults. Certain tumors are more likely to occur in childhood and adolescence, and others are more likely to occur in later life. The basic treatment is essentially the same regardless of the age of the patient.

Treatment is largely dictated by the natural history of the lesion, but the presence of a lesion near a growth plate or the influence of preferred treatment on an epiphysis may be cause for modifying the treatment accordingly. The form of treatment used is also influenced by the surgical accessibility of the lesion, a problem not peculiar to tumors of the pediatric patient. Treatment, therefore, may involve observation of the lesion when the diagnosis is evidenced by roentgenographic and clinical correlation, simple biopsy, excision with or without curettage and bone graft, resection, ablative amputation, radiation, or even cryosurgery.

Bone tumors confront the surgeon with the problem not only of controlling the osseous lesion but also of preserving or restoring useful function. In benign osseous lesions, eradication is usually carried out by excision of the lesion and restoration of the integrity of the bone with autogenous grafts (Figures 1, 2, and 3). Local excision, which is the most conservative of our surgical approaches, preserves the function of the musculoskeletal system and the neighboring joint. This involves radical exteriorization of the bone, often with as much as three-fourths of the circumference of the bone being removed to allow complete visualization of the tumor cavity for excision of the tumor with a curette (Figure 4). However, extensive and recurrent benign osseous lesions require en bloc resection for cure, often with the function in the adjacent joint being sacrificed. After resection, various methods are available to restore the integrity of the limb. Advances are being made in segmental prosthetic replacement of the hip, knee, and shoulder after resection of bone tumors, as well as in allograft replacement. However, in this age group we prefer to use bone-grafting techniques and to achieve a definitive segmental arthrodesis after resection of a benign tumor. (Figure 5).

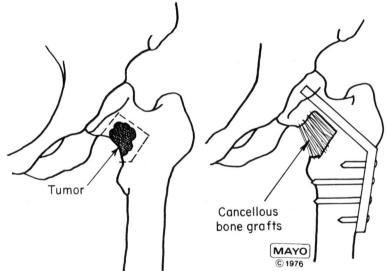

Tumor

Cancellous bone grafts

MAYO
© 1976

Figure 1   Diagram illustrating excision of benign osseous lesion of femoral neck with restoration of integrity of bone with cancellous bone grafts and internal fixation.

TUMORS OF CHONDROGENIC ORIGIN

Osteochondroma (osteocartilaginous exostosis) is the most common benign bone tumor of children and is included in this group because it is formed by progressive enchondral ossification of a growing cartilaginous cap. The cap is attached to a bony stalk (pedunculated) or to a broad base of bone (sessile), commonly in the juxtaepiphyseal region, and the osteocartilaginous exostosis is frequently multiple and often familial (Figure 6).

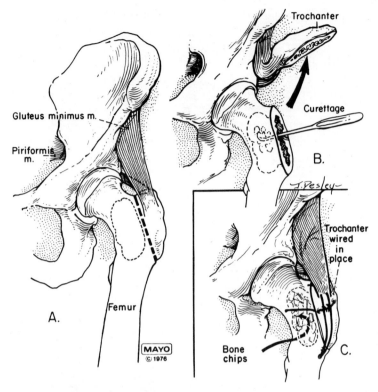

Figure 2 Diagrammatic illustration of curettage and bone grafting of lesion of proximal femur utilizing transtrochanteric approach as a pedicle bone graft. Trochanteric apophysis should be closed when this approach is utilized.

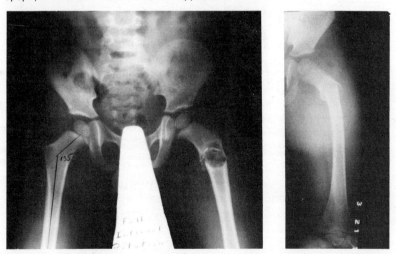

Figure 3 **A** and **B** Anteroposterior and lateral roentgenograms of pelvis and left proximal femur showing unicameral bone cyst with pathologic fracture.

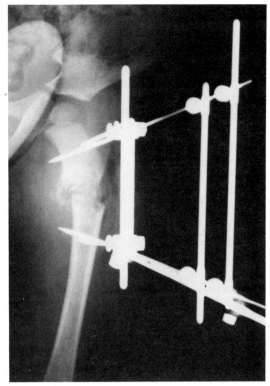

Figure 3   C Anteroposterior roentgenogram of left proximal femur after curettage and bone grafting of cyst, with maintenance of stability and alignment by means of extraskeletal fixation.

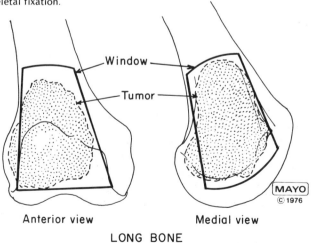

Window

Tumor

MAYO
© 1976

Anterior view   Medial view

LONG BONE

Figure 4   Diagrammatic illustration of radical exteriorization of benign osseous lesion of distal femur to provide direct visualization of the entire tumor cavity for curettage.

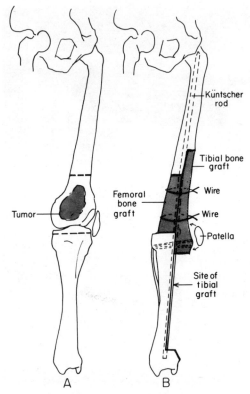

Figure 5. Diagrammatic illustration of segmental arthrodesis using a slide graft from the ipsilateral tibia after resection of the distal femus for a benign osseous lesion.

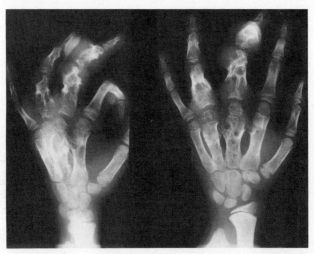

Figure 6. Lateral (**A**) and anteroposterior (**B**) roentgenograms showing multiple chondromatosis in left hand.

Observation is the usual treatment of these lesions, both for solitary or multiple lesions. Removal is indicated only if the lesion is large enough to cause symptoms from mechanical and factitious reasons or is growing disproportionately in size. Occasionally removal is done for cosmetic reasons. Because the incidence of malignant transformation is less than 1%, the routine removal of these tumors is not justified. When necessary, adequate removal involves thorough excision of the base of the exostosis. Occasionally, excision will entail a bone graft, because some of the bases are broad and the bone will be weakened when the exostosis is removed.

Chondroma is a lesion of mature hyaline cartilage occurring either centrally in the bone (enchondroma) or, less frequently, the periosteum (periosteal or juxtacortical chondroma) (Figures 7 and 8). Some of the lesions probably represent failure of normal enchondral ossification, as in Ollier's disease. More than half of the lesions occur in the hands and feet, and 90% occur in the hand. Roentgenographically, the chondroma presents as a well-circumscribed, rarefied tumor, often with stippled or mottled calcification. Histologically, a certain amount of cellular atypia may be present in the periosteal chondroma, in those occuring in the hands and feet, or in those occurring in Ollier's disease (multiple widespread enchondromatosis with a tendency to unilaterality). A related disorder is Maffucci's syndrome, which is characterized by skeletal chondromatosis associated with angiomas of the soft tissues. These two syndromes have been stated to be associated with a high rate of malignant transformation; however, we believe that chondromas, singly or multiply, in the pediatric age group are virtually always benign.

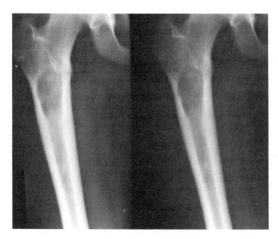

Figure 7. Anteroposterior roentgenograms showing benign enchondroma in right proximal femur in 11-year-old patient.

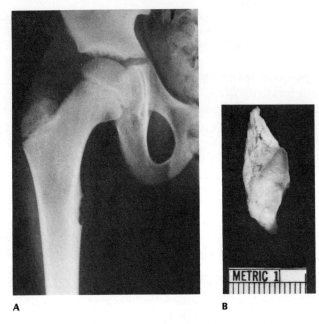

A   B

Figure 8.   **A.** Anteroposterior roentgenogram showing periosteal chondroma in right proximal femur. **B.** Surgical specimen showing typical translucent hyaline cartilage.

Treatment is dictated by the circumstances. Usually, observation is recommended in the case of the benign-appearing asymptomatic lesion that does not structurally weaken the bone. Curettage and filling of the defect by the use of corticocancellous grafts is the course taken when there is a pathologic fracture. This procedure is best done after the fracture has healed and continuity of the bone has been restored. Periosteal chondromas should be excised en bloc.[5] Multiple familial enchondromatosis presents a similar problem in the individual lesions, which become troublesome and must be treated accordingly.

Benign chondroblastoma is a rare lesion; 75% occuring in persons who are in their second decade. First called "calcifying giant cell tumor" by Ewing in 1928, then "epiphyseal chondromatous giant cell tumor" by Codman in 1931, and finally "benign chondroblastoma" by Jaffe and Lichtenstein in 1942, this lesion is usually found in the epiphysis of a long bone in the pediatric age group (Figure 9).[6-8] The tumor, which is considered to arise from "rests" of epiphyseal cartilage, contains zones of chondroid material with well-defined chondroblasts containing round or oval nuclei in a stroma that has an appearance similar to that of the giant cell tumor. The lesion is best treated by excision—often with curettage—and bone grafting. The problem of recurrence, as noted by Dahlin and

Ivins and again by Barnes and associates, have led some to try other methods, including cryosurgery, as advocated by Hickey and Jacobs.[9-11]

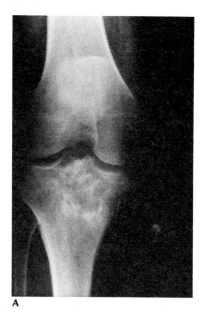
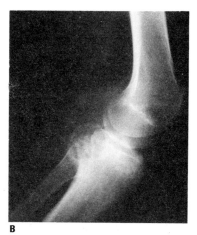

A   B

Figure 9. Anteroposterior (**A**) and lateral (**B**) roentgenograms showing rarefied lesion in proximal tibia situated posteriorly and extending to the articular surface. Flecks of clacification are present in this benign chondroblastoma.

Another recently reported phenomenon is the presence of pulmonary metastases in benign chondroblastoma.[12-15] The metastatic lesions, though like those of benign giant cell tumors which metastasize to the lungs, tend to be nonprogressive and usually are not life-threatening. Radiation for the primary lesion is to be avoided because it may cause malignant transformation of these lesions.

Chondromyxoid fibroma is considered to be very closely related to chondroblastoma. In a comprehensive review by Rahimi et al, slightly less than half of the lesions were found in patients who were less than 20 years old.[16] The lesion is most often located in the metaphyseal region, usually near the epiphysis, and radiographically the lesion most often is seen as an eccentric, well-circumscribed rarefaction with slight sclerotic scalloped margins. Because of a high rate of recurrence after curettage, eradication of the lesion is best accomplished by en bloc resection and bone grafting when possible.[9 16] Radiation therapy is contraindicated.

TUMORS OF OSTEOGENIC ORIGIN

Osteoid osteoma accounts for 10% of benign bone tumors, and 90% of these occur in persons who are from 5 to 20 years old. At least half of the lesions occur in the femur and tibia, but the lesion can occur in any bone and usually is less than 1 cm in size. The nidus of osteoid osteoma consists of a small, usually oval, lucent area surrounded by reactive sclerotic bone (Figures 10 and 11A). Pain is by far the most frequent presenting complaint, and it is often worse at night. Aspirin offers a peculiarly salutary effect by relieving pain.

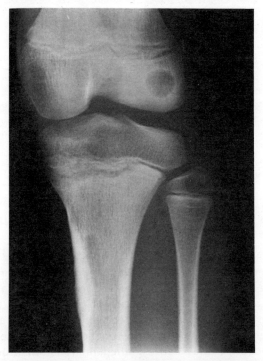

Figure 10. Osteoid osteoma involving the distal femoral epiphysis in 11-year-old boy.

Often the diagnosis is obscure, and considerable skill is needed to demonstrate the lesion roentgenographically after it has become suspected by the characteristic history. The many pitfalls in the diagnosis of osteoid osteoma have been well documented in the recent literature.[17] For example, it may masquerade as an idiopathic scoliosis; in this situation, the main clue to its true nature may be a worsening of the scoliosis when the supine position is assumed.[18] Tomography and angiography have been advocated as helpful in the diagnostic evaluation, the latter showing a circumscribed blush in the early arterial phase which lasts well into the venous phase.[18] [19]

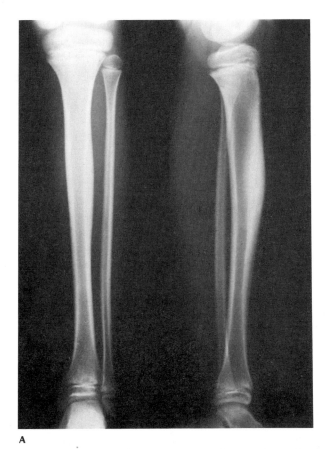

A

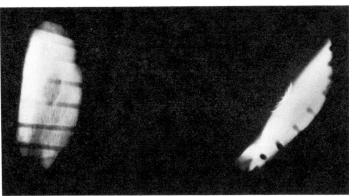

B

Figure 11. **A.** Anteroposterior and lateral roentgenograms of left tibia showing typical osteoid osteoma with lucent central nidus and surrounding reactive cortical sclerosis. **B.** Roentgenograms showing localization of nidus on surgical specimen after excision.

244

Treatment is by surgical excision, and this is best done under roentgenographic control (Figure 11B). The problem of recurrence when removal is inadequate has been well described, and proper identification of the nidus should be made before and after en bloc removal with the use of serial blocks and roentgenograms of the excised bone.[17] [20-22] Curettage is to be discouraged because of the risk of leaving the nidus behind and the difficulty in pathologic diagnosis of the specimen so obtained. Often the defect after excision is large enough to require bone grafting.

Benign osteoblastoma (giant osteoid osteoma) is rarer than the closely related osteoid osteoma, but approximately 70% of them are found in patients who are less than 20 years old. Although the lesion has a similar histologic appearance, it differs from the osteoid osteoma in that it is usually larger, shows a predilection for the spinal column, and does not share as limited a growth potential. Pain is the usual presenting complaint, but neurologic deficits also can be seen, as it is frequently located near the spinal cord and the merging nerve roots (Figure 12). Another recently reported presentation is osteomalacia, which in two patients was reported to be cured by resection of the osteoblastoma.[23] We believe that this lesion has no inherent tendency for spontaneous malignant transformation and agree with Marsh et al that radiation is contraindicated if the lesion is surgically accessible and that complete excision would be ideal, although "cures" have been achieved by curettage alone.[24-26]

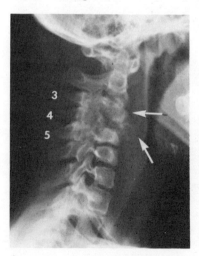 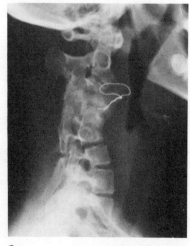

A   B

Figure 12. **A.** Lateral roentgenogram of cervical spinal column in 14-year-old girl showing destruction of fourth cervical vertebra due to osteoblastoma (arrows). This was associated with a quadriparesis. **B.** After excision of lesion and anterior and posterior decompression with anterior cervical fusion, C-2 to C-5.

TUMORS OF FIBROGENIC ORIGIN

Fibroma of bone generally includes nonossifying or nonosteogenic fibroma, metaphyseal fibrous defect (Figure 13), fibrous cortical defect, and "xanthofibroma." Periosteal desmoid is another less cellular variant of these fibrous tumors and may result from trauma.

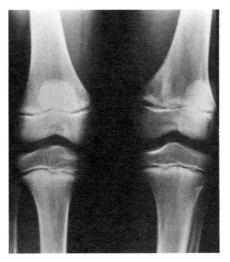
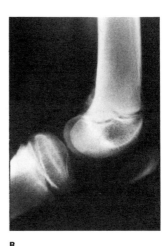

A   **B**

Figure 13. Anteroposterior (**A**) and lateral (**B**) roentgenograms of left knee showing typical metaphyseal fibrous cortical defect.

Fibromas are benign fibroblastic masses occuring in bone almost exclusively in persons who are in their first two decades. The lesion usually arises in the metaphyseal portion of long bones, most frequently in the femur. The lesions are usually asymptomatic and found coincidentally, but they may cause slight swelling or localized pain if large enough. Roentgenograms reveal that the lesion is eccentrically located, often with slight bulging of the cortical outline and a multiloculated appearance.

Treatment of the lesion depends on three factors: the certainty of the diagnosis, the structural integrity of the bone, and the proximity of the lesion to the epiphyseal plate. If the diagnosis is fairly certain by roentgenographic and clinical evidence and the lesion does not threaten the strength of the bone, observation alone is indicated. Otherwise conservative surgery with curettage and bone grafting may be necessary.

Desmoplastic fibroma of bone, as an entity, has been well described in the recent literature.[27] Almost 60% of these lesions are found in the pediatric age group; most commonly they affect the metaphyseal region of long bones. The tumor retains its benign appearance histologically even with multiple recurrences, which are very likely with the lesion. Thus, the preferred treatment is wide resection or thorough curettage, followed by bone grafting and avoidance of radiation or ablative methods of treatment.

TUMORS OF VASCULAR ORIGIN

Hemangioma of bone is a benign vascular tumor that is rare in all age groups and is particularly rare in children. Of the 56 hemangiomas of bone in our series, only 4 were found in patients under 20 years of age.[28] Two closely related syndromes of bone with apparent vascular origin, massive osteolysis and skeletal (cystic) angiomatosis, are more frequently found in these younger age groups. Of 15 patients with cystic angiomatosis whose histories were reviewed by Boyle, only one was over 20 years old.[29] Although histologically these entities are similar to cavernous hemangioma, roentgenographically and clinically they represent destructive and aggressive lesions, which makes treatment difficult. The lesions are often too widespread for effective surgical treatment, and radiation and chemotherapy do not influence the already unpredictable course. The solitary hemangioma is more amenable to conservative therapy, but its infrequence and usually asymptomatic presentation may make this unnecessary.

TUMORS OF UNKNOWN ORIGIN

Benign giant cell tumor of the bone is rare in the child and adolescent, but about 10% occur in this age group. The lesion is composed of osteoclastic multinucleated giant cells and is found in the epiphyseal end of a long bone, eccentrically situated and roentgenographically lytic (Figure 14). Because of its proximity to the end of the long bone, the lesion often presents with joint symptoms. Although spontaneous malignant transformation has been reported, transformation most frequently occurs after radiation therapy.[30] In our experience, irradiation has induced malignant transformation in 20% of patients. Multicentric giant cell tumor of bone has been reported and shows similar sex and age incidences and the same high rate of recurrence after inadequate removal.[31] Giant cell tumor may produce lung metastasis, but like chondroblastoma, the metastatic lesions are histologically benign and usually nonprogressive and not life-threatening.

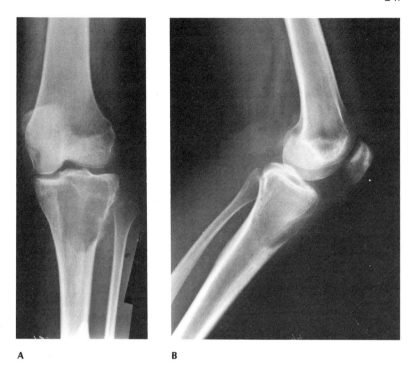

A   B

Figure 14.   Anteroposterior (**A**) and lateral (**B**) roentgenograms of left proximal tibia showing extensive giant cell tumor in femur of 15-year-old boy.

Treatment of the giant cell tumor requires judgment on how adequately to deal with this histologically benign lesion, which is often highly aggressive, frequently recurs, and occasionally shows malignant tranformation. It is one of the most difficult tumors to treat because of its tendency to recur. All of the tumor cells must be removed to effect a cure (Figure 15).

Because the lesion often involves the lower end of the femur or upper end of the tibia, which are important weight-bearing areas, radical surgery presents a problem in regard to function, and overly radical treatment should be avoided. For small intraosseous lesions without a large soft tissue component, radical exteriorization and complete curettage with bone grafting still offer the most reasonable and practical way of treating most of these lesions while preserving function in the neighboring joint. In our hands this method has resulted in a cure rate of approximately 70%. However, extensive lesions with a large soft tissue component or a pathologic fracture require radical en bloc resection for cure. This usually necessitates sacrificing the adjacent joint. Various techniques are available to bridge the defect or replace the joint, depending on the

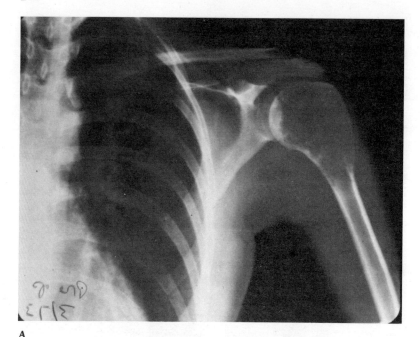

A

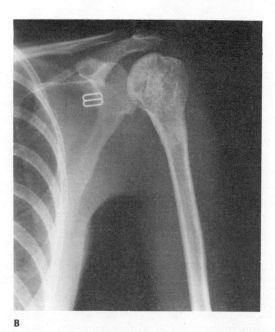

B

Figure 15. **A.** Anteroposterior roentgenogram of left proximal humerus showing extensive destruction from giant cell tumor in 16-year-old boy. **B.** There is no evidence of recurrence 4½ years after radical exteriorization, curettage, and bone grafting.

location of the lesion.[32] Cryosurgery offers some hope, but it is still in the experimental stage and thus far has not been free of articular damage secondary to the freezing.[11] [33]

CONDITIONS SIMULATING BENIGN BONE TUMORS

Unicameral bone cyst is the most common tumorlike affection of bone in adolescent children. It frequently occurs at the upper end of the humerus (Figure 16) but is also found in many other areas. The lesion is referred to as active if it abuts the epiphyseal line, and as latent if it has migrated away from the plate with growth. The roentgenographic findings are those of a fusiform, lytic widening of the bone commonly associated with a pathologic fracture.

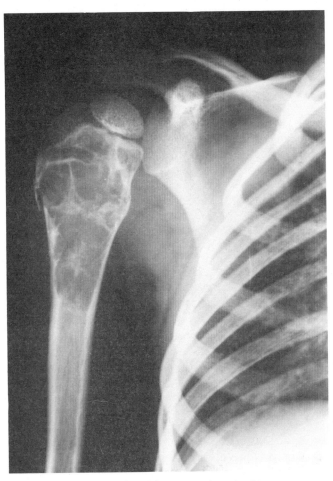

Figure 16. Typical unicameral bone cyst of proximal humerus.

250

Treatment of the lesion ranges from observation, radiation, "implosion" of the cortical walls, simple curettage, and bone grafting to subtotal resection with or without strut bone grafting (Figure 17), with a resultant recurrence rate of 5% to 18%.[34] Recently, Spence et al have reported good results with freeze-dried, crushed cortical bone allograft.[35] They encourage the use of such allografts in order to avoid the morbidity and complications associated with autogenous bone use, and point out the well-known, improved results obtained following complete packing of the lesion with bone graft in children with latent cysts who were more than ten years of age.

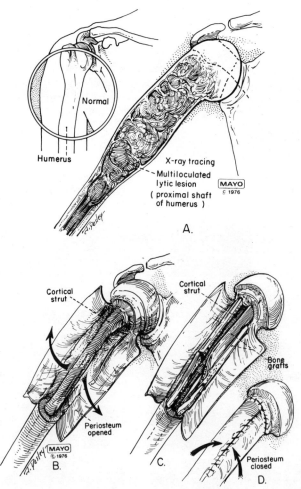

Figure 17 A-D Diagrammatic illustration of unicameral bone cyst and radical exteriorization, with removal of three-fourths of circumferences of the surrounding cortex, followed by curettage and bone grafting.

In our experience, the most practical method is wide exteriorization of the entire cavity with complete curettage of the cyst lining and filling of the cavity with autogenous iliac bone (Figure 18). In the presence of a pathologic fracture, the lesion should be immobilized and the fracture allowed to heal before the lesion is excised and bone grafting is done, particularly if one believes that 15% of these cysts heal after fracture.[36] A recent European report claims good results with aspiration and injection of corticosteroids.[37]

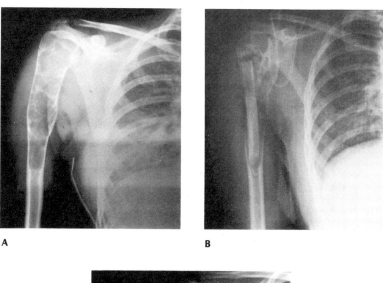

A   B

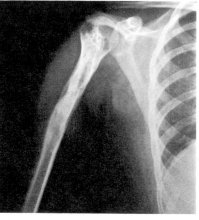

C

Figure 18. **A.** Anteroposterior roentgenogram showing extensive unicameral bone cyst in 15-year-old girl. **B.** After excision and grafting. **C.** Anteroposterior roentgenogram four years after excision and autogenous bone grafting. (Both iliac and tibial bone struts were utilized.)

252

Aneurysmal bone cyst is relatively frequent in childhood: 75% of the lesions occur in patients who are less than 20 years of age.[38] [39] The lesion tends to occur in the metaphysis of long bones or in the vertebrae (Figure 19). Clinically, pain and swelling are frequent presenting complaints. The roentgenographic appearance is characteristic, with an eccentric, well-outlined area of rarefaction often bulging the periosteum and demarcated at the periphery by new bone formation. The high recurrence rate of the lesion has led some authors to recommend more radical forms of treatment, including cryosurgery.[38] [40] We believe that complete surgical excision is the preferred treatment and that curettage and bone grafting should be done when complete en bloc excision is not possible. We recommend that radiation not be used as therapy except when the lesion is in the most surgically inaccessible location. We have no experience with cryosurgery of these lesions.

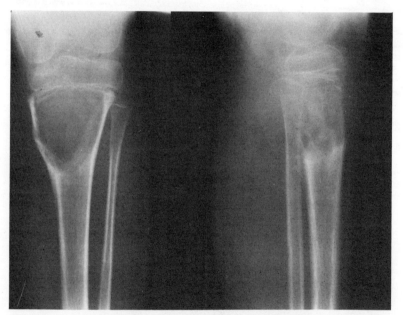

Figure 19. Aneurysmal bone cyst of left metaphyseal region and left proximal tibia in an 11-year-old child. Curettage and bone grafting were performed.

Histiocytosis X simulates a primary bone tumor and most often affects children. This condition includes three syndromes: eosinophilic granuloma, Hand-Schüller-Christian syndrome, and Letterer-Siwe disease—each of which represents different clinical manifestations of the basic disorder of proliferation of histiocytic cells in tissue.[41] [42] The osseous lesions are usually roentgenographically distinct, well-outlined areas of rarefaction which occur singly or multiply and have a predilection for the skull.

Treatment of the osseous lesion is partly dependent on the severity or type of histiocytosis X present. In eosinophilic granuloma and mild Hand-Schüller-Christian disease, low-dosage radiation therapy is employed with good results; in more disseminated disease, steroids, chemotherapy, and occasionally radiotherapy have been used with varying results. The problem of administering radiation to a lesion near an epiphysis has been exaggerated. The dose of radiation needed is generally less than that which can damage the epiphyseal plate.

If located in the vertebral body, the lesion produces a classic coinlike collapse of the vertebral centrum, "vertebra plana." Although while formerly treated with radiation, in recent years the lesion has been observed in the hope that it will heal spontaneously. If the patient is asymptomatic, immobilization alone might be tried before resorting to radiation.

Fibrous dysplasia is relatively common in childhood and adolescence and represents a developmental anomaly of bone formation. The lesion may occur in either monostotic or polystotic form (when the latter is associated with precocious puberty and the presence of café-au-lait spots, it is known as Albright's syndrome). The upper part of the femur is a site frequently affected. Treatment of the lesion is primarily conservative because growth of the dysplasia often ceases with puberty. Occasionally, however, reconstructive surgery is necessary due to deformation of the bone or pathologic fracture. When biopsy for diagnosis is necessary, curettage with bone graft is usually adequate. Radiation therapy is contraindicated because of the high risk of sarcomatous transformation.

SUMMARY

Benign bone tumors of children, and their treatment, present a special challenge, both from a diagnostic and a therapeutic point of view. The tumors themselves take on added significance, in spite of their benign character, because of their possible effect, and the possible effects of therapy, on the growth and development of the bone involved. In addition to recognizing the problems related to growth potential, we must realize the psychologic effects that the tumor (even if benign) and its treatment may have on the patient in this formative time of life. In our experience, a multidisciplinary, team approach to management has done much to facilitate diagnosis and improve the results of treatment.

REFERENCES

1. Dahlin, D.C.: *Bone Tumors: General Aspects and Data on 6,221 Cases.* 3d ed. Springfield, IL, Charles C Thomas, 1978.
2. Hart, J.A.L.: Intraosseous lipoma. *J Bone Joint Surg* [Br] 55:624–632, 1973.
3. Tang, T.T., Zuege, R.C., Babbitt, D.P. et al: Angioglomoid tumor of bone: a case report. *J Bone Joint Surg* [Am] 58:873–876, 1976.
4. Wirth, W.A. and Bray, C.B., Jr.: Intra-osseous neurilemoma: case report and review of thirty-one cases from the literature. *J Bone Joint Surg* [Am] 59:252–255, 1977.
5. Rockwell, M.A. Saiter, E.T., and Enneking, W.F.: Periosteal chondroma. *J Bone Joint Surg* [Am] 54:102–108, 1972.
6. Ewing, J., cited by Huvos, A.G., Marcove, R.C., Erlandson, R.A. et al: Chondroblastoma of bone: a clinicopathologic and electron microscopic study. *Cancer* 29:760–771, 1972.
7. Codman, E.A.: Epiphyseal chondromatous giant cell tumors of the upper end of the humerus. *Surg Gynecol Obstet* 52:543–548, 1931.
8. Jaffe, H.L. and Lichtenstein, L.: Benign chondroblastoma of bone: a reinterpretation of the so-called calcifying or chondromatous giant cell tumor. *Am J Pathol* 18:969–991, 1942.
9. Dahlin, D.C. and Ivins, J.C.: Benign chondroblastoma: a study of 125 cases. *Cancer* 30:401–413, 1972.
10. Barnes, S.N., Calandruccio, R.A., Pitcock, J.A. et al: Chondroblastoma of bone: complications and problems, abstracted. *J Bone Joint Surg* [Am] 58:734, 1976.
11. Hickey, C.H. and Jacobs, P.A.: Experience with closed cryosurgical techniques. Read before the Symposium on Bone Tumor Therapy Choices, Milwaukee, WI, November 17 and 18, 1977.
12. Green, P. and Whittaker, R.P.: Benign chondroblastoma: case report with pulmonary metastasis. *J Bone Joint Surg* [Am] 57:418–420, 1975.
13. Riddell, R.J., Louis, C.J. and Bromberger, N.A.: Pulmonary metastases from chondroblastoma of the tibia: report of a case. *J Bone Joint Surg* [Br] 55:848–853, 1973.
14. Schajowicz, F. and Gallardo, H.: Epiphysial chondroblastoma of bone: a clinicopathological study of sixty-nine cases. *J Bone Joint Surg* [Br] 52:205–226, 1970.
15. Sweetnam, R. and Ross, K.: Surgical treatment of pulmonary metastases from primary tumours of bone. *J Bone Joint Surg* [Br] 49:74–79, 1967.
16. Rahimi, A., Beabout, J.W., Ivins, J.C. et al: Chondromyxoid

fibroma: a clinicopathologic study of 76 cases. *Cancer* 30:726-736, 1972.

17. Sim, F.H., Dahlin, D.C., and Beabout, J.W.: Osteoid-osteoma: diagnostic problems. *J Bone Joint Surg* [Am] 57:154-159, 1975.

18. Keim, H.A. and Reina, E.G.: Osteoidosteoma as a cause of scoliosis. *J Bone Joint Surg* [Am] 57:159-163, 1975.

19. O'Hara, J.P., Tegtmeyer, C., Sweet, D.E. et al: Angiography in the diagnosis of osteoidosteoma of the hand. *J Bone Joint Surg* [Am] 57:163-166, 1975.

20. Worland, R.L., Ryder, C.T., and Johnston, A.D.: Recurrent osteoidosteoma: report of a case. *J Bone Joint Surg* [Am] 57:277-278, 1975.

21. Worrall, V.T., III and Ferguson, R.: Osteoidosteoma in childhood, abstracted. *J Bone Joint Surg* [Am] 57:1026, 1975.

22. Ponseti, I. and Barta, C.K.: Osteoidosteoma. *J Bone Joint Burg* 29:767-776, 1947.

23. Yoshikawa, S., Nakamura, T., Takagi, M. et al: Benign osteoblastoma as a cause of osteomalacia: a report of two cases. *J Bone Joint Surg* [Br] 59:279-286, 1977.

24. Schajowicz, F. and Lemos, C.: Malignant osteoblastoma. *J Bone Joint Surg* [Br] 58:202-211, 1976.

25. Seki, T., Fukuda, H., Ishii, Y. et al: Malignant transformation of benign osteoblastoma: a case report. *J Bone Joint Surg* [Am] 57:424-436, 1975.

26. Marsh, B.W., Bonfiglio, M., Brady, L.P. et al: Benign osteoblastoma: range of manifestations. *J Bone Joint Surg* [Am] 57:1-9, 1975.

27. Sugiura, I.: Desmoplastic fibroma: case report and review of the literature. *J Bone Joint Surg* [Am] 58:126-130, 1976.

28. Unni, K.K., Ivins, J.C., Beabout, J.W. et al: Hemangioma, hemangiopericytoma, and hemangioendothelioma (angiosarcoma) of bone. *Cancer* 27:1403-1414, 1971.

29. Boyle, W.J.: Cystic angiomatosis of bone: a report of three cases and review of the literature. *J Bone Joint Surg* [Br] 54:626-636, 1972.

30. Larsson, S-E., Lorentzon, R., and Boquist, L.: Giant cell tumor of bone: a demographic, clinical, and histopathological study of all cases recorded in the Swedish Cancer Registry for the years 1958 through 1968. *J Bone Joint Surg* [Am] 57:167-173, 1975.

31. Sim, F.H., Dahlin, D.C., and Beabout, J.W.: Multicentric giant cell tumor of bone. *J Bone Joint Surg* [Am] 59:1052-1060, 1977.

32. Enneking, W.F., and Shirley, P.D.: Resection-arthrodesis for malignant and potentially malignant lesions about the knee using an

intramedullary rod and local bone grafts. *J Bone Joint Surg* [Am] 59:223–236, 1977.

33. Marcove, R.C., Lyden, J.P., Huvos, A.G. et al: Giant cell tumors treated by cryosurgery: a report of twenty-five cases. *J Bone Joint Surg* [Am] 55:1633–1644, 1973.

34. McCay, D.W. and Nason, S.S.: Treatment of unicameral bone cysts by subtotal resection without grafts. *J Bone Joint Surg* [Am] 59:515–519, 1977.

35. Spence, K.F., Jr., Bright, R.W., Fitzgerald, S.P. et al: Solitary unicameral bone cyst: treatment with freeze-dried, crushed cortical bone allograft: a review of 144 cases. *J Bone Joint Surg* [Am] 58:636–641, 1976.

36. Spjut, H.J., Dorfman, H.D., Fechner, R.E. et al: Tumors of bone and cartilage. Atlas of Tumor Pathology, 2nd series, fascicle 5. Armed Forces Institute of Pathology, Washington, D.C., 1971, pp 329–330, 352.

37. Campanacci, M., DeSessa, L., and Bellando-Randone, P.: Bone cysts: review of 275 cases. Results of surgical treatment and early results of treatment by methylprehnisolone acetate injections. *Chir Organi Mov* 62:471–482, 1976.

38. Biesecker, J.L., Marcove, R.C., Huvos, A.G. et al: Aneurysmal bone cysts: a clinicopathologic study of sixty-six cases. *Cancer* 26:615–625, 1970.

39. Buraczewski, J. and Dabska, M.: Pathogenesis of aneurysmal bone cyst: relationship between the aneurysmal bone cyst and fibrous dysplasia of bone. *Cancer* 28:597–604, 1971.

40. Ruiter, D.J., van Rijssel, T.G., and van der Velde, E.A.: Aneurysmal bone cysts: a clinicopathological study of 105 cases. *Cancer* 39:2231–2239, 1977.

41. Enriquez, P., Dahlin, D.C., Hayles, A.B. et al: Histiocytosis X: a clinical study. *Mayo Clin Proc* 42:88–99, 1967.

42. Schajowicz, F. and Slullitel, J.: Eosinophilic granuloma of bone and its relationship to Hand-Schüller-Christian and Letterer-Siwe syndromes. *J Bone Joint Surg* [Br] 55:545–565, 1973.

17 Psychosocial Aspects of the Treatment of Bone Tumors in Children and Adolescents

Antoinette L. Pieroni, A.C.S.W.

1. The patient and his or her family
2. Special problems related to therapy
3. Role of the social worker

The word "tumor" usually means "cancer," even to the medically unsophisticated person, and the word "cancer" usually means a long, debilitating illness ending in death. Since bone tumors most often affect adolescents, this age group is of special interest in regard to the psychosocial problems such diseases impose.

Adolescence—that period in life between the naiveté of childhood and the awareness and responsibility of adulthood—is fraught with difficulties even for the healthy child. Physical and attitudinal changes are significant and frequent. Muscles and breasts develop; voices change pitch. Intellectual changes may be less obvious, but the opinion of parents and other adults are questioned as the adolescent seeks to establish his independence in this sphere. Social change is also great. Competition can be keen and pressures intense. Conforming to one's peers—acting, dressing, and talking like them—and being liked and accepted by them, lend security. Routine and ritual are important.

During this period the adolescent most needs respect and acceptance from the adult world. Parents often forget, though, what they thought or felt as adolescents. Even worse, they may try to use their children to compensate for perceived shortcomings of their own youth, and thus add to their children's difficulties in growing up.

THE PATIENT AND HIS OR HER FAMILY

A diagnosis of cancer compounds all the problems of adolescence and changes the patient and his family immediately. There is severe shock — the often unintelligible words used to describe the condition and its treatment, fear of the unknown, and the threat of death disorganize them. The adolescent is afraid he will be different and wonders *how* different. What will he be able to do, and how will he look? Perhaps he will have to be hospitalized — if so, will he become isolated from his friends and family? His fears and frustrations will often be translated into anger at the people who will treat him. He will resent the fact that he confided his symptoms to his parents, as this eventually led to the discovery of the cancer. He will be angry at them for subjecting him to all that is going on. He will be angry, too, at his siblings and friends for being able to do things he fears he may no longer be able to do. His fear that he will die or that he will be alone will frighten and haunt him. Circumstances will demand that he show maturity beyond his years.

The parents also experience emotional turmoil. Their first reaction is denial. They think: "This cannot be true"; "There must be a mistake"; "We want another opinion." They feel isolated and think themselves to be the only parents to face this tragedy. They see their child as already dead, and this is silently reinforced by relatives and friends who are also frightened. Anger at the world, at God — even at their child — filters through, and depression sets in.

When the diagnosis is discussed for the first time, it is of the utmost importance that the physician sit down with the family in a quiet, comfortable, private room and explain everything honestly and gently in words they can understand. The physician should begin with the diagnosis and what the diagnosis means. He should then explain what treatment is planned and what its effects and side effects will be. A frank and honest discussion is necessary, for what is to be conveyed is a realistic hope for a good prognosis. This first interview gives the parents an opportunity to ask questions, and it allows them and the physician to begin to know each other. The parents must first understand the diagnosis themselves if they are to be able to help their child. The adolescent should also receive an honest explanation of the diagnosis of his condition and of the treatment that is planned and how it will affect him.

The patient's and his family's acceptance of the diagnosis, and their adaptation to treatment, can be helped by all the members of the medical team. The team members must deal honestly with the patient and his family, and they must be dedicated to giving emotional support as well as expert therapy. It is particularly important that each member of the medical team, starting with the physician, comes to know the adolescent well—that he is familiar with his life-style, his hobbies, his ambitions, and his fears. In this way the medical team may help the parents to reinforce the patient's strengths.

Rarely can the fears and feelings of the family be dealt with until their worries about practical problems have been taken care of. For instance, there are the general, mundane problems which face every family in such a situation—such as finding a suitable place to stay near the hospital if they come from a distance; arranging for the care of other family members while one or both parents are away from home; and finding financial resources, if these are needed, for the medical care.

A significant problem affecting the adolescent and his parents is that of his education. The patient may have a hospital teacher while he is in the hospital so that he can keep up with his studies and also have something to look forward to and gain a feeling of accomplishment. Later, a home tutor from his school district can help him until he is ready to return to school. Experience has also shown that reentering the classroom is made more tolerable if the patient, his parents, and a member of the medical team can prepare the school and the patient's classmates for his return by supplying them with some knowledge of his illness, of changes in his physical appearance, and of limitations on his activities.

Other problems that can and do come up are: where to obtain a prosthesis; where to find recreation for both the patient and his family; how to fill a father's time profitably while he stays with his child in the hospital and away from his home and work? Patients and their parents are ready to discuss their anxieties and emotions once some of these pressing practical problems have been taken care of.

SPECIAL PROBLEMS RELATED TO THERAPY

The hospital environment is a frightening one in itself, and the three modes of treatment usually employed for children with sarcomas—surgery, radiation therapy, and chemotherapy—add to the general anxiety aroused.

Surgery is probably the most familiar of these therapies to the general public. Most patients facing surgery consider the operating room a frightening unknown, and like anyone else, the adolescent who must undergo surgery may fear anesthesia because it means a loss of awareness and control over his situation. When surgery involves amputation of a limb, however, fears and anxieties increase. Patients with osteosarcoma are those most likely to be confronted with the necessity for surgery, and they may fear castration, the reactions of their peers to their changed appearance, and death. They may also be anxious about what will become of the removed limb and the possibility of phantom pains. These special concerns of the young cancer patient should be anticipated and his fears and questions responded to with emotional support, factual information on the operation and what he can expect afterward, and assurances of continued help in adjusting and coping later on.

Radiation therapy, with its hard tables and gigantic machinery, and its invisible rays that heal, combines elements of a horror room with the mystical. As is surgery, the whole process is very difficult to comprehend, and it would be helpful if hospitals would conduct tours of anesthesia rooms and recovery and radiation therapy rooms so that the patient and his parents could become acquainted with these "unknowns," and so that questions concerning various aspects of the facilities could be answered beforehand to alleviate much of the fear.

Chemotherapy produces varying emotional and physical reactions. Oral medication is acceptable. Medication by the intravenous route, however, is more frightening and traumatic. By whatever method, though, cancer chemotherapy is a completely new experience for the adolescent. He vomits violently; he needs to be monitored closely for mouth sores and other side effects; he starts losing his hair; he wonders what the drugs are doing to his body and to his mind.

Alopecia is one of the most traumatic side effects of cancer therapy. Adolescent girls have confided to the author that losing their hair was worse than losing their limb. Help in obtaining a wig or hairpiece is very important, but first the patient has to get used to the idea of wearing one. Knowing that the hair loss is temporary is of little comfort initially, and this attitude must be treated with honesty and understanding by the entire medical team.

All of these effects contribute to a drastic change in the adolescent's self-concept as therapy proceeds. He will say: "I am different;" "people are staring;" "my friends will feel sorry for me." Indeed, many aspects of cancer therapy set the patient apart. For example, radiation therapists may use indelible skin markers to define radiation therapy portals, and most teenage girls will ask, "How can I wear a bikini if I have ugly marks on my skin?" The adolescent patient may also feel isolated from his peers because he is faced with the reality of his own mortality, and they have not yet been confronted by this fact.

A great deal of time must be spent by the chemotherapist, psychiatrist, surgeon, radiation therapist, social worker, and other members of the team in getting to know the child and in explaining to him and to his family the side effects of the various modes of his total therapy. It takes much patience and time to help a family not to despair over their child's feelings of isolation. They need to help him develop other activities which involve his friends. Alex's case serves as a good example.

> When he was 13, Alex had a forequarter amputation of his left arm. Within one year after his operation, he was helped to turn his denial and anger toward positive goals. Alex took second place in both tennis and golf tournaments for his age group in his section of the state. Today he is married, has two children, and is counseling handicapped patients. Much time was spent over the years to help his parents allow Alex to establish his independence.*

Interpersonal relationships are usually difficult. Teenagers constantly test the people around them. They become angry and depressed when plans for the future are disrupted by the medication schedule. It is extremely difficult, but not impossible—with the help of tutors and with a great deal of support from everyone involved (family and medical personnel)—for the patient to manage high school work during the course of treatment. It *is* almost impossible to pursue university studies, and many patients feel they lose two years of their youth. However, with help and support from the medical team and family members, these years need not be a total loss, and the patient should be encouraged to undertake something he or she can handle until something such as college attendance is feasible. Laurie's case provides a good example.

> Although Laurie had to postpone her college education, she was able to tutor young children with learning disabilities, and she felt she was contributing to their lives and to society.*

For the older adolescent who is of working age, the period of treatment can be a disaster. No employer will hire a person who is sick one out of every three weeks. It is this group of patients that is the most angry and depressed and that feels the most isolated. They and their families need a great deal of guidance and counseling, and

*Antoinette Pieroni 1965; unpublished data.

possibly referral to appropriate community agencies.

Loss of self-esteem and changes in body image exaggerate the problems of interpersonal peer relationships, so that making friends, dating, and marriage may not seem possible. Patients who fear that sexual intercourse may be impossible or that they might become sterile must be helped to overcome their fears, and their parents and the parents of their friends must also be educated in this regard. Since multidisciplinary therapy has allowed more children to survive malignant disease, more former patients have married and had children of their own, and for the most part lead normal lives. Such individuals may be invited to speak with other patients who fear they may be excluded from these experiences.

We are learning from former patients that other problems— such as job discrimination, even when there is no visible handicap; obstacles to obtaining life and health insurance; and automatic exclusion from military service—may arise many years after treatment. These former patients and their families need to know that they will receive continued support from the medical and social work staffs. Indeed, we encourage the family to bring friends to key people in the community to visit and talk with the medical team at any time, because this broader involvement benefits the patient and his family.

ROLE OF THE SOCIAL WORKER

The social worker plays a key role in all of the relationships between the patient and family, and the medical team. If at all possible, the social worker should be present at the first interview between the physician and the patient and his family—at the very least, the social worker must be introduced to the family very soon thereafter. As a member of the medical team, the social worker can ensure that the patient and his family understand the procedures outlined and can reinforce what has been explained by the physician. It is the social worker who becomes acquainted with the personalities of all the members of the family and with the family's socioeconomic status, which plays an important role in the overall emotional situation.

The social worker learns of the stresses and crises which have occurred previously and how the family has coped with them. From this information, strengths and weaknesses of the family situation are learned and the social worker can make an assessment of how the family may meet the present crisis. He or she acts as liaison between the family and the hospital and should bring to the team his or her own special skills of interviewing and casework, knowledge of interpersonal dynamics, and access to resources in the community.

He or she can help ensure good mental health—from the first interview through treatment and recovery, or on to what may be the terminal stage and the grieving period which follows.

A good relationship must be established in the first interview. A useful technique is to begin to know the family by obtaining basic, factual information, such as names, ages, and school grades of other children; employment and income of the parents; and the housing situation. Listening to tones of voice, watching mannerisms, and being aware of hesitancies are just as important as obtaining facts. During this interview, the social worker attempts to clarify any misconceptions which the patient and parents may have received from the first medical interview, and asks, "What did the doctor tell you?" "What did you understand?" The social worker learns from the parents about the patient's personality, what he knows about his diagnosis, what else he has heard, and what thoughts he has expressed. The social worker is then able to help the family through the initial period of crisis by making suggestions for coping, by giving continuous support, and most importantly, by passing relevant information on to the physician and other team members involved in the patient's care.

It is also important for the social worker to be sensitive to the ethnic, cultural, educational, attitudinal, and emotional differences of each family and to any changes that may occur throughout the period. This means that the social worker must constantly adjust his or her management of each family situation.

The method the social worker most often uses to help patients and families is the one-to-one interview, which puts a person more at ease in talking about anxieties, feelings, and family problems. A second method is that of family interviews, at which both parents, and sometimes the patient and/or siblings, are present. Families need help in achieving self-awareness. They need a great deal of emotional support to function effectively, and it is very important to get siblings involved. They have to be told what is going on so that normal life can continue and guilt can be minimized. They should be encouraged to go to the hospital or outpatient facility, where they can learn about the illness and its treatment firsthand, within the limits of their understanding. This also helps diminish any fears they may have about developing illness themselves.

Parent groups have become more popular and are used to great advantage. The parents gain much support from each other and feel less isolated. They can communicate with each other more easily than they can with the professionals involved. They are not afraid to discuss any subject—whether it be good nutrition, marital problems, or facing the death of their child—because they know they all

264

share the same crises. They help each other with practical problems by providing transportation and sharing meals, and they offer each other true friendship.

Group sessions have been so successful that a new kind of group has been formed by those parents who have lost a child. They continue to lend each other support and are now directing their energies toward service-oriented projects such as volunteering, transporting other patients to the clinic, baby-sitting for patients' siblings, obtaining blood, and organizing fund drives to help parents whose children are still under treatment.

CONCLUSIONS

Current therapy may prolong a child's life, but that life may not be worth living if concern with the quality of that life is not uppermost in our minds. Each member of the team has his or her particular skill to bring to the task of improving the quality of the patient's life and of the life of each member of his family. Team members may even include such nonprofessionals as the ward maid or the parking lot attendant, who, with a kind word at a crucial moment, can do much to offer the support a family needs.

In helping patients, either by prolonging life or by providing support and understanding in the terminal stage of illness, we must be honest—both factually and emotionally—with ourselves, and with our patients and their families. We must understand our patients as individuals and we must respect them. When a good relationship has been formed and the family trusts the oncology team, they will be able to accept the diagnosis. Treatment then becomes tolerable. We can do our best only if we are honest, concerned, and sincere.

SUGGESTED READING

Burton, L.: The Family Life of Sick Children. Routledge & Kegan Paul, Boston, 1975.

Buscaglia, L.: The Disabled and Their Parents: A Counselling Challenge. Charles B. Slack, Inc., Thorofare, NJ, 1975.

Dunphy, J.E.: Annual discourse: on caring for the patient with cancer. N Engl J Med 295:313–319, 1975.

Feifel, H. (ed): The Meaning of Death. McGraw-Hill, Inc., New York, 1959.

Friedman, S.B.: Psychological aspects of sudden unexpected death in infants and children. Pediatr Clin North Am 25:103–111, 1974.

Godenne, G.H.: The masked signs of adolescent depression. *Med Insight* 6:9-11, 1974.

Held, M.L.: The dying child: the importance of understanding. *Med Insight* 6:13-17, 1974.

Josselyn, I.M.: *The Adolescent and His World.* Family Service Association of America, New York, 1952.

Leichtman, S.R. and Friedman, S.B.: Social and psychological development of adolescents and the relationship to chronic illness. *Med Clin North Am* 59:1319-1328, 1975.

Lewis, M.: *Clinical Aspects of Child Development.* Lea & Febiger, Philadelphia, 1971.

Moos, R.H. (ed): *Coping with Physical Illness.* Plenum Press, New York, 1977.

Parad, H. (ed): *Crisis Intervention: Selected Readings.* Family Service Association of America, New York, 1952.

Spinetta, J.J.: The child with cancer: patterns of communication. Read before the 57th Annual Meeting of the Western Psychological Association, Seattle, WA, April 22, 1977.